# Bodily Chronicles: The Science of Being Human

Daniel Alvarez Yeomans
Franz Gerhard Enkerlin Lozano
Juan Pedro Silva Martinez

The wise adapt themselves to circumstances, as water molds itself to the pitcher.

## Caffeine: The World's Favorite Stimulant and Its Impact on Our Bodies

Caffeine, consumed annually in quantities equivalent to 14 Eiffel Towers in weight, is more than just a popular beverage ingredient; it's the most widely used drug globally. Found in coffee, tea, some sodas, chocolate, and even in products labeled decaf, caffeine is renowned for enhancing alertness, focus, and energy levels, especially when sleep is lacking. However, its effects extend beyond a mere energy boost, influencing blood pressure and anxiety levels.

Originally evolved in plants as a defense mechanism against insects and a memory aid in nectar, caffeine's role in the human body is quite different. It acts as a stimulant for the central nervous system, keeping us awake by impeding the function of adenosine, a key sleep-inducing molecule. As the body breaks down ATP for energy, it releases adenosine, which, upon binding to neural receptors, slows neuron activity, leading to sleepiness. Caffeine, resembling adenosine's structure, blocks these receptors without activating them, thus inhibiting the inhibitor – stimulating rather than sedating.

Caffeine's impact extends to our emotions as well. It interacts with adenosine receptors linked to dopamine receptors, influencing feelings of pleasure. By blocking adenosine's access, caffeine allows dopamine to function more freely, enhancing mood.

Long-term benefits of caffeine have also been observed, potentially reducing the risk of Parkinson's, Alzheimer's, and certain cancers.

Athletically, caffeine's ability to increase fat burning has led to its scrutiny in competitive sports, with limits imposed on its consumption in events like the Olympics. However, caffeine's effects are not universally positive. It can raise heart rate and blood pressure, cause gastrointestinal issues, and contribute to insomnia and anxiety. Additionally, the body's adaptation to regular caffeine intake can lead to increased tolerance and withdrawal symptoms upon cessation.

Despite these mixed effects, caffeine remains a staple in many diets. Its widespread consumption and varied impacts make it a fascinating subject for study and discussion. As we continue to enjoy our favorite caffeinated beverages, understanding caffeine's complex role in our bodies helps us appreciate this ubiquitous stimulant's full spectrum of effects.

## Understanding Our Body's Need for Movement

In our modern lifestyle, the act of sitting for extended periods has become a norm, but it's far from what our bodies are designed for. Contrary to the comfort we feel while sitting, our bodies are silently protesting, longing for movement. This video explores why our bodies are built to move and the consequences of a sedentary lifestyle.

The human body, with its 360 joints and about 700 skeletal muscles, is structured for fluid and easy motion. Our upright posture against gravity, blood circulation, nerve cell function, and skin elasticity all hint at a design meant for regular movement.

So, what happens when we defy this innate design and remain seated for too long? The spine, our literal backbone, suffers from prolonged sitting, especially in a slumped posture. This position leads to uneven pressure on the spine, causing wear and tear on spinal discs, straining ligaments and muscles, and reducing lung capacity.

Sitting affects not only our skeletal structure but also our soft tissues. Extended sitting compresses nerves, arteries, and veins, leading to numbness, swelling, and reduced blood flow. Moreover, sitting deactivates essential enzymes like lipoprotein lipase, which breaks down fats in the blood, thereby impacting our fat metabolism.

The brain, too, feels the impact of prolonged sitting. Reduced blood flow and oxygen supply due to inactivity can lead to decreased concentration and slowed brain function. But the implications of a sedentary lifestyle extend beyond temporary discomforts.

Recent studies have linked long periods of sitting with increased risks of certain cancers, heart disease, and contributing factors to diabetes, kidney, and liver problems. Inactivity is estimated to cause 9% of premature deaths worldwide annually – over 5 million lives.

This video urges a reevaluation of our sitting habits. Simple changes, like maintaining a straighter spine when we must sit and taking frequent breaks to move around, can mitigate the risks associated with prolonged sitting. It reminds us that our bodies are fundamentally designed for motion, not for stillness, and our health depends on honoring this design.

## The language of sleep: Dreams

Since the third millennium BCE, when Mesopotamian kings inscribed their dreams on wax tablets, humanity has been fascinated with the world of dreams. This fascination continued a thousand years later with the ancient Egyptians, who compiled a dream book cataloging over a hundred dreams and their meanings. Centuries have passed, yet our quest to decipher the mysteries of dreams persists, evolving alongside scientific and technological advancements.

Sigmund Freud, in the early 1900s, proposed a compelling theory: dreams are the fulfillment of our subconscious wishes. He believed that our dreams, including nightmares, are symbolic manifestations of our unconscious thoughts, urges, and desires. Freud argued that the analysis of these symbols could reveal hidden psychological issues and aid in their resolution.

Another intriguing theory suggests that we dream to remember. A study in 2010 demonstrated that subjects navigating a complex 3D maze performed significantly better if they had dreamt about the maze. This finding suggests that certain memory processes might only occur during sleep, with dreams being an indicator of these processes.

Conversely, the 1983 neurobiological theory of reverse learning posits that we dream to forget. It argues that during REM sleep, our neocortex reviews and discards redundant neural connections, preventing our brains from being overwhelmed by unnecessary thoughts.

The continual activation theory offers a different perspective: dreams are a result of our brain's need to constantly consolidate and create long-term memories for proper functioning. When external stimuli are low, such as in sleep, the brain generates data from memory, which manifests as dreams.

The primitive instinct rehearsal theory delves into dreams of danger and threat. It suggests that these dreams serve as a rehearsal for our fight-or-flight responses, keeping these instincts sharp for real-life scenarios. This theory extends to all instincts, suggesting that dreams can be a practice ground for various survival skills.

Dreams might also play a role in psychological healing. During the REM stage of sleep, stress neurotransmitters are less active, even during dreams of traumatic events. This reduced stress level could allow for a clearer perspective and healthier psychological processing of traumatic experiences.

Solving problems through dreams is another fascinating aspect. Dreams allow the mind to transcend the constraints of reality and conventional logic, creating limitless scenarios to grasp and solve problems. This concept is exemplified by August Kekulé, whose dream about the structure of the benzene molecule led to a scientific breakthrough.

These theories, each unique and compelling, reflect our evolving understanding of the complex world of dreams. As technology advances, we inch closer to unraveling the definitive purpose of dreaming. Until then, the journey through the enigmatic and captivating landscape of our dreams continues, offering insights, mysteries, and endless possibilities for exploration.

## The Liver Punch: Anatomy of a Knockout

The liver, a seemingly robust organ, holds a peculiar vulnerability – a well-placed punch to this area can incapacitate even the toughest of individuals. This phenomenon isn't just about experiencing pain; it's a systemic shutdown orchestrated by the body's innate response to trauma.

If you've never felt the searing agony of a liver shot, consider yourself lucky. The liver, situated on the right side of the body below the diaphragm, is not just another organ. It's a critical player in detoxification, protein synthesis, and digestion, and it's the largest and heaviest internal organ, weighing about 1.5 kilograms in an adult.

A direct punch to the liver, be it from a fist, knee, or kick, triggers an excruciating response. This isn't just about physical toughness or willpower; a precise strike to the liver can shut down your body, leaving you breathless, fatigued, and possibly collapsed on the ground.

This reaction to a liver shot starkly contrasts with a blow to the head. While a head shot may disorient and not immediately register pain, a liver shot leaves the mind clear but the body incapacitated. Delving deeper into the liver's structure reveals why this is so.

The liver's wedge shape, pliability, and nerve-rich capsule make it particularly susceptible to impact. When struck, pressure changes within the liver stimulate nerve fibers linked to the autonomic

nervous system (ANS). This triggers a cascade of events, starting with the stimulation of the vagus nerve.

This stimulation causes blood vessels to dilate, except in the brain, and simultaneously slows the heart rate. This combination of events leads to a dramatic drop in blood pressure. The body's response, an attempt to redirect blood flow to the brain, is to collapse into a horizontal position. In severe cases, this shock to the system can even cause unconsciousness.

In professional fighting, factors like pain, stress, and dehydration exacerbate this response. Interestingly, while other internal organs can respond similarly to trauma, the liver's size and position make it more vulnerable. It protrudes slightly from under the rib cage, unlike the more protected kidneys, surrounded by muscle and nestled within the ribcage.

The evolutionary trajectory of the human body, with the liver growing in importance and size, raises questions about why the rib cage didn't adapt to offer more protection to this vital organ. Despite this vulnerability, the human body remains a marvel of nature, not a perfect system.

The takeaway is clear: a liver punch is a powerful tool in combat sports, capable of turning the tide in a fight. It serves as a reminder of our body's complex responses to trauma and the delicate balance it maintains under stress. So, the next time you witness a fighter crumble from a liver shot, remember the intricate physiological ballet unfolding within.

## The Opioid Crisis: A Journey from Ancient Remedies to Modern Epidemic

Over 3,000 years ago, the ancient Egyptians and Minoans discovered the dual nature of a particular flower – its capacity to induce pleasure and alleviate pain. This flower, the source of opium, marked the beginning of humanity's intricate relationship with opioids. Fast forward to the 19th century, and morphine, a key compound of opium, was isolated, heralding a new era in medical pain management.

Morphine, codeine, and other derivatives from the poppy plant are termed opiates. The 20th century saw the development of synthetic substances akin to these opiates, including heroin, hydrocodone, oxycodone, and fentanyl, collectively known as opioids. These substances, whether natural or synthetic, legal or illicit, are potent painkillers but come with a high risk of addiction.

In the 1980s and 90s, aggressive marketing by pharmaceutical companies downplayed the addictive potential of opioid painkillers, leading to a surge in prescriptions and, subsequently, cases of addiction, sparking a crisis that persists today.

To comprehend the addictive nature of opioids, it's crucial to understand their impact on the human body, from initial use to long-term effects and the consequences of cessation. All opioids, regardless of their specific chemistry, act on the brain's opioid receptors, which are also the binding sites for endorphins. Opioids bind more strongly and for longer durations than endorphins, managing more severe pain.

Opioid receptors control not only pain but also mood and various bodily functions. When opioids bind to these receptors, they trigger dopamine release, leading to feelings of pleasure and the euphoria often associated with opioid highs. Additionally, opioids suppress noradrenaline production, affecting wakefulness, breathing, digestion, and blood pressure. Excessive doses can dangerously lower heart and breathing rates, potentially leading to unconsciousness or death.

The body develops tolerance to opioids over time, necessitating higher doses to achieve the same effects, a pathway to physical dependence and addiction. Increased opioid use can significantly suppress noradrenaline levels, affecting basic bodily functions. The body compensates by increasing noradrenaline receptor sensitivity, becoming dependent on opioids to maintain this new balance.

Abrupt cessation of opioid use disrupts this balance, leading to a surge in noradrenaline levels but with an abundance of overly sensitive receptors, resulting in severe withdrawal symptoms.

The opioid crisis has evolved over decades. Initially, middle-aged individuals became addicted to prescribed painkillers, but now younger people are increasingly exposed to opioids, often transitioning from prescription drugs to cheaper, illicit alternatives like heroin or synthetic opioids.

In combating this crisis, naloxone has emerged as a crucial tool against overdose, as it can block and reverse opioid effects on the brain. However, opioid addiction is complex, often intertwined with mental health issues, necessitating comprehensive treatment approaches that combine medication, health services, and psychotherapy. Yet, access to these programs is hindered by high costs, long waiting lists, and the requirement of complete detoxification before treatment.

Opioid maintenance programs offer an alternative, using drugs like methadone and buprenorphine to avoid withdrawal symptoms while preventing the psychoactive effects of opioids. However, prescribing these maintenance drugs requires special waivers, contrasting the ease of prescribing opioid painkillers.

The path forward in addressing the opioid epidemic is challenging, filled with the need for better resources, understanding, and access to treatment options. From its ancient origins to its modern implications, the journey of opioids reflects a complex interplay of medicine, addiction, and societal impact.

## The Bilingual Brain: Unraveling the Linguistic Mosaic

In the diversity of human communication, if you find yourself resonating with 'Ja', 'Oui', or "Si", and are absorbing this in English, you're likely a part of the global bilingual or multilingual majority. This linguistic diversity isn't just a passport to easier travels or enjoying films without subtitles; it signifies that your brain might operate distinctly compared to monolingual individuals.

Understanding a language encompasses active skills like speaking, writing and passive ones like listening and reading. While a balanced bilingual might have comparable proficiency in all aspects of two languages, the reality for most bilinguals is a mix of varying degrees of mastery in each language.

Consider Gabriela, a young girl whose family moved from Peru to the U.S. when she was two. She represents a compound bilingual, developing two linguistic codes simultaneously, intertwining English and Spanish as she interprets her world. Her teenage brother might be a coordinated bilingual, learning English academically while maintaining Spanish for home and social interactions. Their parents, likely subordinate bilinguals, learn English through the lens of their native Spanish.

To the outside world, these distinctions in bilingualism are subtle. However, recent advancements in brain imaging have offered insights into how bilingualism shapes the brain. The left hemisphere, typically dominant in logic and analytics, contrasts with the right's prowess in emotional and social processing. Language, involving both realms, is influenced by this lateralization, which evolves with age.

This leads us to the critical period hypothesis, suggesting that children, with their highly plastic brains, can use both hemispheres for language acquisition, providing a more nuanced grasp of social and emotional contexts. Adults, on the other hand, tend to lateralize language to one hemisphere, usually the left.

Adult language learners often approach a second language with less emotional bias and a more rational perspective. Regardless of the age at which additional languages are acquired, multilingualism confers notable brain benefits. These include increased density of gray matter and heightened activity in certain brain regions when using a second language.

The bilingual brain enjoys a rigorous workout throughout life, potentially delaying Alzheimer's and dementia onset by up to five years. This understanding marks a significant shift from past views where bilingualism was mistakenly seen as a developmental hindrance.

Recent studies have shown that while bilingual individuals may experience increased reaction times and errors in cross-language contexts, the mental effort in switching between languages enhances the dorsolateral prefrontal cortex, a key
player in executive functions, problem-solving, and task switching.
Thus, bilingualism might not directly equate to being smarter, but it certainly fosters a healthier, more complex, and engaged brain. For those who haven't had the opportunity to learn a second language early in life, it's never too late to embrace the linguistic leap from 'hello' to 'hallo', 'bonjour', or 'olá'. In the realm of brain health, even a small dose of linguistic exercise can have far-reaching benefits.

## The Enigma of Longevity: Aging

In 1997, the world witnessed the end of an extraordinary life. Jean Calment, a French woman, closed her eyes for the last time after 122 years and 164 days, setting a record as the oldest known person. Her remarkable age inspired a millionaire to offer $1 million to anyone who could surpass her lifespan. But the reality of achieving such longevity is a complex and elusive endeavor.

The human body is not engineered for extreme aging. Our biological design seems to cap our lifespan at around 90 years. But what exactly does aging entail? How does it interfere with our body's innate struggle to survive?

Aging, in its essence, represents the culmination of both intrinsic bodily processes and environmental interactions. Factors like sunlight and airborne toxins gradually induce changes in our body's molecular and cellular structures, leading to functional decline and, ultimately, the organism's failure.

Scientists are just beginning to unravel the mechanisms behind aging, identifying nine key physiological traits that play a pivotal role, ranging from genetic mutations to a decline in cellular regeneration.

One critical aspect is the accumulation of genetic damage over time. DNA lesions, both in dividing and non-dividing cells, especially in mitochondria, the powerhouses of the cell, contribute to this deterioration. As mitochondrial function declines,
 so does the vitality of cells and organs.
Epigenetic alterations, changes in gene expression patterns, also mark the aging process. Genes that are dormant in youth become active in old age, potentially leading to degenerative diseases like Alzheimer's.
Even our body's natural regenerative processes cannot outpace the effects of aging. Telomeres, protective caps at the ends of chromosomes, shorten with each cell division, eventually leading to cell death and impeding the body's renewal abilities.
Cell senescence, another facet of aging, acts as a double-edged sword. While it prevents cancerous cell proliferation, it also inhibits healthy cell growth, diminishing the body's regenerative capacity.
Stem cells, vital for tissue renewal, also succumb to the effects of aging. With time, they diminish in number and lose their regenerative potential, impacting the maintenance of organ functions.
Other cellular functions also decline with age, including protein quality control and intercellular communication. This deterioration affects overall metabolic activity and the body's operational efficiency.

The quest to understand aging raises profound questions. Can lifestyle choices like diet and exercise significantly extend our lifespan? Will future technologies, such as gene therapy or nanobots, artificially prolong our years? And, perhaps most intriguingly, do we genuinely desire
a life span that exceeds our current biological limits?
Jean Calment's 122 years stand as a beacon of human potential, igniting curiosity and ambition in the quest for longevity. Her life is not just a record to be broken but a testament to the enigmatic and fascinating journey of human aging.

# A Revolution in Reproduction: The IVF Story

In 1978, a landmark event in medical history unfolded when Louise Brown, the first baby conceived through in vitro fertilization (IVF), was born. This moment marked a revolutionary leap in reproductive medicine, addressing the challenges faced by one in eight heterosexual couples struggling with infertility, alongside homosexual couples and single parents seeking clinical assistance in childbearing.

IVF, now a common practice, has led to the birth of over five million babies. This technology mirrors the marvel of sexual reproduction. To grasp IVF's intricacies, we must first explore the natural process of conception, beginning in an unlikely place: the brain.

The journey of baby-making commences about 15 days before fertilization, with the anterior pituitary gland releasing follicle-stimulating hormone (FSH). This hormone ripens ovarian follicles, each harboring an egg, and stimulates estrogen release. Typically, only one follicle fully matures, signaling its readiness through rising estrogen levels.

When estrogen peaks, the pituitary gland releases a surge of luteinizing hormone (LH), triggering ovulation and the release of the egg. The egg's journey then leads it to the fallopian tube, aided by the fimbriae's delicate guidance.

The egg, the body's largest cell, is encased in a zona pellucida, a protective shell ensuring only one sperm, the smallest cell, can fertilize it. From the over a hundred million sperm released during intercourse, only a handful reach the egg, and just one breaches the zona pellucida to achieve fertilization.

Following fertilization, the zygote evolves into an embryo, journeying towards the uterus for implantation. The embryo's implantation stimulates hormonal signals, maintaining the corpus luteum, which produces progesterone crucial for sustaining early pregnancy.

Now, transitioning to baby-making in the lab: IVF begins with administering FSH to stimulate the ovaries into producing multiple eggs. These eggs are retrieved under anesthesia, while sperm samples are typically obtained through masturbation.

In the lab, the eggs are prepared for fertilization. Fertilization can occur naturally with sperm incubation or through intracytoplasmic sperm injection (ICSI), where a single sperm is injected into the egg, beneficial in cases of poor sperm quality.

After fertilization, embryos undergo genetic screening, can be frozen for future use, or transferred into the uterus using a catheter. The embryos are typically transferred either three days post-fertilization, at the eight-cell stage, or five days post-fertilization, at the blastocyst stage.

In scenarios of poor egg quality, donor eggs or a gestational carrier may be employed. To enhance success rates, which peak at 40% for women
under 35, multiple embryos are sometimes transferred, leading to higher incidences of twins or triplets compared to natural pregnancies.
Millions of babies, like Louise Brown, have been born healthy through IVF. The long-term impacts of ovarian stimulation remain under study, but IVF is generally considered safe. With advancements in genetic testing, delayed childbearing, and decreasing costs, the future may see artificial reproduction methods like IVF becoming more prevalent than natural conception. This narrative isn't just a tale of scientific triumph; it's a story of hope, possibilities, and the ever-evolving journey of human reproduction.

## The Unseen Impact: Understanding Concussions in Sports

In the United States, the world of sports and recreational activities is a vibrant tapestry of enthusiasm and skill, but beneath this surface lies a concerning reality. Each year, between 2.5 and 4 million concussions occur, raising critical questions about their impact on the brain.

The brain, a soft, fatty organ akin to jello, resides within the skull's protective embrace. Under normal circumstances, this setup serves well, but a sudden jolt can disrupt this harmony, causing the brain to collide with the skull's hard interior. This is where the complexity of a concussion begins.

Unlike jello, the brain comprises an intricate network of 90 billion neurons, each connected by slender, fragile axons. These axons, vital for signal transmission and bodily control, are vulnerable to damage upon impact. When they stretch or tear, the ensuing chaos is not just a temporary disruption in communication. The damaged axons degenerate, releasing toxins and leading to further neuronal death.

This cascade of events is what we call a concussion. Its manifestations are varied and personal, ranging from headaches and blurred vision to altered mood and cognitive difficulties. The diversity in symptoms is a reflection of each brain's unique makeup and response to injury. Fortunately, most concussions heal with time, given sufficient rest and a gradual return to normal activities. The myth of avoiding sleep post-concussion is just that—a myth unless a more severe brain injury is suspected.

However, concussions are not always straightforward. Post-concussion syndrome (PCS) can emerge, prolonging symptoms like headaches and cognitive difficulties, affecting personal relationships and quality of life for months or even years. Returning to sports too soon or ignoring a concussion increases the risk of developing PCS.

Subconcussive impacts, though less severe than concussions, pose a hidden danger. These repeated, minor jolts can lead to serious conditions over time. Soccer players, frequently heading balls, offer a glimpse into this risk. Research using diffusion tensor imaging has shown that repeated heading can damage the structural integrity of axon bundles, akin to the fraying of a rope, and correlate with memory performance issues.

These subconcussive hits can accumulate, leading to chronic traumatic encephalopathy (CTE), a degenerative brain disease manifesting in mood and behavioral changes, cognitive decline, and potentially dementia. The underlying mechanism involves tau proteins, which usually support axonal structure. Repeated impacts disrupt these proteins, causing them to clump together and impair neuronal function. This damage can progress even after the head impacts
have ceased.

Alarmingly, a significant percentage of concussions in sports, especially in football, go unreported and untreated. This may be due to difficulty recognizing a concussion or pressure to continue playing despite injuries. This culture not only hinders recovery but poses a grave risk.

The narrative of concussions in sports is a tale of unseen dangers and misunderstood injuries. It's a call to acknowledge the vulnerability of our brains and the need for better protection and care in the athletic world. As we advance in understanding concussions, it becomes imperative to prioritize the health and safety of athletes, ensuring the longevity of both their careers and cognitive well-being.

## Sisters' Puzzle: DNA and Ancestry

Two sisters, intertwined by blood and history, embarked on a journey of genetic discovery. They shared the same home, the same laughter, the same parents. Yet, when they delved into the world of DNA testing, the results unveiled a curious riddle: one sister was shown to be 10% French, the other, not a trace.

This is not just about numbers, but the intricate tapestry of our genetic inheritance. Our DNA, the blueprint of our being, holds secrets, but also limitations in its revelations. It's a story that tells us more about probabilities and past recombination than definitive ancestral origins.

Within each of us, lies a vast universe of about 6 billion base pairs, a labyrinth of genetic information. But in this vastness, 99% is a shared journey of humankind, a common story. It's in the scarce 1% where our individual ancestral stories are whispered.

The sisters' divergence stems from this unique realm. Each chromosome, a beacon of heritage from each parent, undergoes a dance of recombination before conception. This dance is a blend of randomness and history, making each sibling's genetic makeup a unique mosaic, a distinctive mix from the same set of ancestors.

The notion of being "French," or any nationality, in genetic terms, is more about representation than lineage. The tests don't trace direct lines to specific ancestors who walked the streets of

France. Instead, they draw comparisons to the genetic markers prevalent in modern French populations, making assumptions based on probabilities and patterns.

But this story has deeper layers. The database of human genomes, predominantly European, paints an incomplete picture, leaving many ancestral voices unheard. The sisters' results are shaped not just by their DNA, but by the stories that are available to be told through the existing database.

As they delve further back, they encounter the ancient chapters of human history, finding echoes of Neanderthal ancestry. This surprising twist reveals the interwoven paths of different species, a testament to our shared evolutionary journey.

Their story is a reminder that our genetic heritage is a complex, ever-changing narrative, shaped by the past, but also by the knowledge and tools we have in the present. The sisters' DNA results, though different, are not contradictions but parallel tales in the vast, unfolding story of human ancestry.

In this journey, the sisters learn that DNA can reveal much, but not everything. It speaks in probabilities and patterns, not certainties. Their quest for understanding their roots teaches them about the beauty of diversity, the intricacy of genetics, and the limitations of our current scientific grasp. The tale of the two sisters and their DNA is a modern parable, a reminder of our interconnected, yet unique, human experience.

## Visionary Craft: The Journey from Keratomileusis to LASIK

In the heart of 1948's bustling medical innovations, a Spanish ophthalmologist, José Ignacio Baracar Moner, stood at the forefront of a revolution. Tired of the constraints of glasses, he dreamt of a world where the eye could be mended from within, liberated from external aids. His ambition was not just a mere fancy; it was a fervent quest to redefine vision correction.

Baracar's method, though radical, was a dance of precision and audacity. He would delicately slice off the front of a patient's cornea, only to plunge it into the icy grip of liquid nitrogen. In his hands, a miniature lathe transformed this frozen disc into a lens of perfect curvature, meticulously crafted to refocus vision. The thawed cornea, now a testament to his skill, was sutured back, a reborn lens offering clarity where there was once blur.

He christened this method 'keratomileusis', a term born from the ancient Greek essence of carving and cornea. Grisly in its conception, yet its results spoke of unwavering reliability.

But how did this procedure intertwine with the intricate workings of the human eye? Keratomileusis was a ballet, correcting the refractive errors that marred the eye's ability to focus light. In myopia, where the world blurs at a distance, or hyperopia, where the far becomes clear while the near dissolves into obscurity, Baracar's method offered a remedy. Even astigmatism, with its dueling curvatures within a single cornea, found a potential resolution under his watchful eye.

As time marched on, the world of eye surgery evolved, embracing the gentler yet equally potent power of lasers. Surgeons now sculpt corneas with the precision of artists, wielding eczema lasers capable of etching the finest details onto a strand of human hair. The process, swift and precise, reshapes the cornea in situ, a dance of light and tissue that culminates in LASIK – a term that echoes its predecessor yet stands as a beacon of modern medical marvel.

And still, the journey of vision correction sails forward. Techniques like SMILE and Laser Blended Vision not only correct errors but also restore the fading sight of aging eyes. With each pulse of the laser, each careful adjustment, we edge closer to Baracar's dream: a world where glasses are relics of the past, and clear vision is but a laser away.

In this dance of light and vision, we find ourselves awash in tears – not of sorrow, but of life. Our eyes, ever-producing tears, remind us of the fluidity and resilience of our sight. In the tale of Baracar's legacy, we find not just the evolution of a medical procedure, but a testament to human ingenuity's endless pursuit to improve, refine, and perfect.

## Illuminating the Mind: The Quest to Understand the Human Brain

In the vast expanse of our solar system, the human brain stands out as the only entity sophisticated enough to study itself. Yet, this self-exploration is a formidable challenge. The brain, a complex organ shielded by the skull and swathed in protective tissue, comprises billions of interconnected cells. This complexity makes understanding diseases like Alzheimer's a daunting task. So, how do we study living brains without causing harm? The answer lies in a trio of innovative techniques: EEG, fMRI, and PET.

Firstly, EEG, or electroencephalography, measures the brain's electrical activity. As brain cells communicate, they generate electrical waves, which are captured by electrodes placed on the skull. EEG has been instrumental in diagnosing conditions like epilepsy and sleep disorders and in exploring brain activity during learning and attention. Its strengths lie in its non-invasiveness, affordability, and speed, capturing changes in mere milliseconds. However, EEG's Achilles' heel is its inability to pinpoint the exact origins of electrical patterns within the brain.

To complement EEG's temporal precision, functional magnetic resonance imaging, or fMRI, steps in. MRI tracks the consumption of oxygen by brain cells, revealing active brain regions. This technique has enabled us to probe into various cognitive and emotional processes, offering

spatial resolution down to a few millimeters. However, fMRI's temporal resolution is significantly slower than EEG's.

The third technique, positron emission tomography or PET, offers even greater precision. PET scans involve injecting a trace amount of radioactive material into the bloodstream and monitoring its movement through the brain. By tailoring the tracer to bind to specific molecules, PET scans can unravel the brain's intricate chemistry, proving invaluable in studying drug effects and detecting diseases like Alzheimer's. Despite its precision, PET's limitation lies in its low time resolution.

These techniques collectively empower doctors and scientists to correlate brain activity with behavior. However, they also underscore our limited understanding of the brain. For instance, in studying memory, researchers might identify active brain regions in fMRI scans but would need further research to unravel the specifics of each region's role and their collaborative functions.

The future of brain imaging promises more advanced technology, potentially capable of distinguishing individual neuronal activity. Until then, our brains continue to measure, analyze, and innovate, relentlessly pursuing the understanding of one of the most remarkable entities we've ever encountered – the human brain itself.

## Traumatic Storm: Understanding and Addressing PTSD

Trauma is a universal human experience, yet its aftermath varies greatly among individuals. While some emerge seemingly unscathed, millions find themselves ensnared by lingering symptoms that disrupt daily life. This condition, known as post-traumatic stress disorder (PTSD), is not a sign of weakness but a treatable malfunction of the body's natural response to danger.

PTSD can stem from a myriad of traumatic events, ranging from personal losses to physical or emotional abuse, accidents, or natural disasters. These experiences can trigger the brain's alarm system, the fight, flight, freeze response, activating the hypothalamic-pituitary-adrenal (HPA) axis. This response mobilizes the autonomic nervous system, flooding the body with stress hormones and preparing it for immediate action.

Even after a traumatic event has passed, elevated stress hormone levels can persist, manifesting as jitteriness, nightmares, and other symptoms. For most, these reactions subside within days or weeks as hormone levels stabilize. However, for some, the symptoms persist or reemerge, leading to PTSD.

The exact mechanisms of PTSD in the brain are not fully understood, but it's believed that continuous activation of the fight-flight-freeze response, possibly due to cortisol, impairs overall brain functioning. Symptoms of PTSD often fall into four categories: intrusive thoughts, avoidance behaviors, negative thoughts and feelings, and reactive symptoms. The intensity and combination of these symptoms vary, and PTSD is typically diagnosed when problems persist for over a month.

Factors like genetics, ongoing stress, and pre-existing mental health conditions can influence the likelihood of developing PTSD. One of the major challenges for those with PTSD is sensitivity to triggers—everyday stimuli that evoke memories of the trauma, reigniting the neurochemical cascade and emotional turmoil of the original event.

Avoiding these triggers can lead to isolation, exacerbating feelings of alienation and misunderstanding. However, there are effective treatments available. Psychotherapy can help patients understand and manage their triggers, while medications and self-care practices like mindfulness and exercise can alleviate symptoms.

Support from friends and family is crucial. Acceptance, empathy, and belief in the person's experiences are key to aiding recovery. Encouraging professional evaluation and treatment can also be immensely helpful.

PTSD, often termed the 'hidden wound', lacks outward physical signs but is a significant mental health challenge. It's a disorder that may be invisible, but it doesn't have to be endured in silence. Understanding and addressing PTSD is vital, not just for those suffering but for society's collective empathy and awareness of mental health issues.

## Steroids: The Unsung Heroes in Medicine's Arsenal

Steroids, often mired in controversy due to their association with sports doping, play a far more diverse and crucial role in medicine than many realize. They are key ingredients in inhalers, creams for treating skin conditions, and injections to reduce inflammation. The steroids used in these medical applications are fundamentally different from those known for muscle building.

To understand why there are so many different types of steroids, it's essential to recognize that the term 'steroid' refers to a specific molecular structure rather than a uniform effect on the body. Steroids, whether naturally occurring or synthetic, share a molecular backbone: four rings consisting of 17 carbon atoms arranged in three hexagons and one pentagon. This structure is the defining characteristic of a steroid, though most also have side chains that significantly influence their function.

The name 'steroid' is derived from cholesterol, a fatty molecule from which our bodies synthesize steroids. This cholesterol base enables steroids to cross cell membranes and directly influence gene expression and protein synthesis within cells. This mechanism differs from many other signaling molecules that cannot penetrate the cell membrane and must exert their effects externally through more complex pathways.

Focusing on anti-inflammatory medications, these are based on cortisol, a naturally occurring steroid and the body's primary stress signal. Cortisol plays a multifaceted role in our body's response to stress, ranging from psychological stress to physical threats like infections or low blood sugar. The brain signals the adrenal glands to release cortisol, which then triggers various physiological responses, including increased glucose production, suppression of non-essential functions like digestion, and activation of the fight, flight, or freeze response.

Cortisol's interaction with the immune system is complex. It can modulate immune functions, increasing or decreasing them depending on the situation. In the context of infection, cortisol suppresses the immune system's inflammatory response, which is beneficial in the short term. However, prolonged exposure to high cortisol levels can weaken the immune system's regenerative capabilities.

Medicinal corticosteroids harness cortisol's immune-modulating effects to combat allergic reactions, rashes, and asthma, all of which are forms of inflammation. These synthetic steroids enhance the body's cortisol supply, thereby dampening hyperactive immune responses. They can enter cells and suppress the genes responsible for inflammatory signals.

The application of steroids varies depending on the condition and the form of the medication.

Inhalers and creams target specific organs like the skin or lungs, while intravenous or oral steroids, used for chronic autoimmune conditions, have a systemic effect. In autoimmune diseases, where the immune system mistakenly attacks the body's own cells, a low dose of steroids can help regulate this misguided immune response.

However, due to the adverse effects of long-term steroid use, higher doses are typically reserved for acute emergencies and flare-ups. Conditions like asthma, poison ivy rashes, and inflammatory bowel disease, seemingly unrelated, share a common thread: an overactive immune response that does more harm than good. Corticosteroids, while not muscle-building, are vital in managing these conditions by tempering the body's defense mechanisms against itself.

In exploring the role of steroids in medicine, we uncover a narrative of complexity and versatility, highlighting their critical function in managing a range of health conditions and offering a deeper understanding of these often misunderstood compounds.

## The Antibiotic Paradox: Navigating the Crisis of Resistance

Antibiotics, the unsung heroes of modern medicine, have quietly underpinned much of our medical progress. They not only cure infectious diseases but also make surgeries, chemotherapy, and organ transplants safer. However, we stand on the brink of losing this crucial ally. Antibiotics are chemicals that inhibit bacterial growth, but alarmingly, some bacteria have developed resistance to all existing antibiotics. Meanwhile, the discovery of new antibiotics has stalled. Yet, there's still hope to turn the tide.

The journey into this predicament began with the discovery of penicillin in 1928 by Alexander Fleming. In his 1945 Nobel Prize acceptance speech, Fleming presciently warned of the potential for bacterial resistance to render antibiotics ineffective. His fears materialized quickly, with resistant bacteria emerging as early as the 1940s and 50s.

Initially, pharmaceutical companies responded by discovering many new antibiotics, a venture both successful and profitable. However, over time, the landscape changed. Newly discovered antibiotics were often effective against a narrower range of infections, making them less profitable. Additionally, the overprescription of antibiotics, including for viral infections, led to increased scrutiny and reduced sales.

Simultaneously, the pharmaceutical industry shifted focus to developing drugs for chronic conditions, which were more profitable due to their long-term usage. By the mid-1980s, no new chemical classes of antibiotics had been discovered, but bacterial resistance continued to grow, facilitated by the sharing of genetic information among bacteria.

Today, multi-drug-resistant bacteria are increasingly common, and some strains are resistant to all our current drugs. The challenge now is to control the use of existing antibiotics, develop new ones, combat resistance, and explore alternative methods to fight bacterial infections.

A significant contributor to antibiotic resistance is agriculture, where antibiotics are used not only to treat infections but also to promote animal growth. This widespread use accelerates the development of resistance, which can then be transferred to humans through the food chain and international trade.

In the quest for new antibiotics, nature offers promising compounds. Microbes and fungi, having evolved in competitive environments, often possess antibiotic properties. Additionally, packaging antibiotics with molecules that inhibit resistance mechanisms, using phages (viruses that target bacteria), and developing vaccines for common infections are promising strategies.

However, the biggest hurdle is funding. Antibiotics are not profitable, leading many pharmaceutical companies to abandon their development. Even

successful new antibiotics struggle to be financially viable. Innovative funding models, like the UK's antibiotic subscription program, are being tested, but global efforts need to be significantly ramped up.

The antibiotic crisis is a paradox of success and failure. While antibiotics have saved countless lives, their overuse and the slow pace of new discoveries have led to a resistance crisis. With enough investment and controlled use of current drugs, we can still overcome this challenge. Just as the accidental discovery of penicillin revolutionized medicine, our response to this crisis could shape the future of healthcare.

## Marijuana and the Mind: Unraveling the Complexities of Cannabis

In 1970, marijuana was cast into the shadows of illegality in the United States, classified as a Schedule 1 drug with no recognized medical uses. This stringent categorization stifled research into its mechanisms and effects for decades. Today, however, the landscape has shifted dramatically. The therapeutic benefits of marijuana are increasingly acknowledged, leading to its legalization for medical use in various nations. Yet, amidst this growing acceptance, a critical question lingers: Is recreational marijuana use detrimental to your brain?

Marijuana's interaction with the body is complex. It acts on the cannabinoid system, which is intricately woven throughout the brain and body. This system, still not fully understood, is influenced by endocannabinoids, molecules native to the body. These endocannabinoids travel in a unique manner, moving backward to provide feedback to the sending neuron, suggesting that the endocannabinoid system's primary role is to modulate other signals.

Marijuana contains two main active compounds: tetrahydrocannabinol (THC) and cannabidiol (CBD). THC is linked to marijuana's psychoactive effects, while CBD is associated with its non-psychoactive impacts. Unlike endocannabinoids, which are released in response to specific stimuli, THC binds to cannabinoid receptors throughout

the brain indiscriminately. This widespread activity, coupled with the system's indirect influence on various other systems, means that marijuana's effects are highly individualized, shaped by each person's unique brain chemistry, genetics, and life experiences.

The potential harmful effects of marijuana, if any, vary significantly from person to person. However, certain risk factors can heighten the likelihood of experiencing negative outcomes. Age is a critical factor. In individuals under 25, cannabinoid receptors are more densely packed in the white matter, which plays a crucial role in communication, learning, memory, and emotions. Frequent marijuana use during this developmental phase can disrupt the formation of white matter tracks and hinder the brain's capacity to form new connections, potentially impairing long-term learning and problem-solving abilities.

Marijuana can also induce hallucinations or paranoid delusions, known as marijuana-induced psychosis. While these symptoms typically recede with cessation of use, they can occasionally reveal a persistent psychotic disorder, particularly in individuals with a family history of such conditions.

Another aspect to consider is the brain's adaptability. With repeated use, the brain becomes less sensitive to marijuana, necessitating higher doses to achieve the same effects. Fortunately, marijuana does not pose a risk of fatal overdose, and withdrawal symptoms, though present, are not as severe or life-threatening as those associated with many other drugs.

So, is marijuana bad for your brain? The answer is nuanced and highly individual. While some risk factors are identifiable, others remain elusive, leaving a margin of uncertainty regarding its potential negative effects. As research continues to peel back the layers of marijuana's impact on the mind, it becomes increasingly clear that its role is as complex as the human brain itself.

In a world where caffeine reigns as the most widely used drug, the quest to understand the substances that influence our minds and bodies is more relevant than ever. For a deeper dive into how another popular substance, caffeine, affects us, further exploration is just a video away.

**The Vicious Cycle of Insomnia: Understanding and Overcoming Sleepless Nights**

What keeps you up at night? Is it the thrill of an upcoming adventure, the weight of unfinished tasks, or perhaps the anxiety of a looming social event? For many, such stress is a fleeting shadow, dissipating as quickly as it appears. But imagine if the very source of your wakefulness was the fear of not sleeping. This paradoxical dilemma is the essence of insomnia, the most prevalent sleep disorder in the world.

Insomnia often starts with mundane disturbances – a partner's snoring, physical discomfort, or emotional stress. Even severe sleep disruptions like jet lag can upset your biological clock, leading to temporary sleep issues. Typically, sleep deprivation is a transient state, with exhaustion eventually claiming victory. However, chronic conditions such as respiratory or gastrointestinal issues can defy this natural resolution, leading to prolonged periods of wakefulness.

As these sleepless nights accumulate, the bedroom, once a sanctuary of rest, becomes a theater of anxiety and restlessness. For insomniacs, the approach of bedtime is met with stress, triggering a cascade of physiological responses. The body floods with stress hormones like cortisol, ramping up heart rate and blood pressure, thrusting the body into a state of hyperarousal.

In this heightened state, the brain becomes hyper-
vigilant, amplifying every minor discomfort and sound, making sleep elusive. When sleep does come, it's often fragmented and unrefreshing. Our brain, which relies on cerebral glucose for energy, normally conserves this resource during healthy sleep. However, in insomniacs, the persistent adrenaline rush accelerates metabolism, depleting the brain's energy reserves and leading to a state of exhaustion upon waking.

This cycle of poor sleep and daytime stress, if prolonged for several months, is diagnosed as chronic insomnia. Interestingly, the biochemical pathways of insomnia share similarities with those of anxiety and depression, suggesting a link among these conditions.

Breaking the cycle of insomnia involves managing the stress that leads to hyperarousal and adopting good sleep practices. Creating a conducive sleep environment, engaging in relaxing activities before bed, and maintaining a consistent sleep schedule can help reorient the body's circadian rhythm.

While some medications can aid sleep, they are not universally effective and can be addictive. It's also crucial to correctly diagnose the cause of sleeplessness. For instance, about 8% of chronic insomnia patients actually suffer from delayed sleep phase disorder (DSPD), where their circadian rhythm is longer than 24 hours, leading to a misalignment with conventional sleep times.

Maintaining a balanced sleep-wake cycle is essential for our physical and mental well-being.

Investing time and effort in a stable bedtime routine is key, but it's important not to let the pursuit of perfect sleep become a source of additional stress. Remember, the journey to a peaceful night's sleep is as much about understanding the nature of insomnia as it is about finding the right solutions.

## The Ever-Changing Battle: Inside the Annual Flu Vaccine Race

In a relentless pursuit of health, researchers across the globe embark on an annual quest, gathering samples from flu patients in a coordinated effort to outsmart one of nature's most adaptable adversaries: the influenza virus. This story isn't just about creating a vaccine; it's a race against time and evolution.

Why, you might ask, do we need a new flu vaccine every year? Unlike diseases like mumps and rubella, where a couple of shots offer a lifetime of protection, the flu presents a unique challenge. The influenza virus is not only diverse, with over 100 subtypes, but it also possesses a remarkable ability to mutate rapidly.

The flu virus operates by hijacking a host's cells, turning them into factories churning out copies of itself. Unlike most viruses, the flu's genetic material is RNA, not DNA. This distinction is crucial. DNA replication in cells comes with a proofreading mechanism, correcting errors. RNA lacks this failsafe, allowing mutations to accumulate and new virus variants to emerge.

This rapid mutation poses a significant problem for vaccine development. Vaccines work by training the immune system to recognize specific antigens, the unique substances on a virus's surface. When the immune system encounters these antigens, it produces antibodies, preparing it to fight off the actual virus. However, due to the flu's rapid mutation, these surface antigens can change, rendering previously effective antibodies less efficient.

Complicating matters further, flu strains can merge, creating new hybrid viruses. This constant evolution makes targeting the flu virus akin to hitting a moving, ever-transforming target. To combat this, scientists tirelessly monitor flu strains worldwide, analyzing data to track mutations and predict which strains will be most prevalent. The World Health Organization convenes experts biannually, once for each hemisphere, to decide which strains should be included in the upcoming season's vaccine. Typically, four strains are selected for the quadrivalent vaccine.

Despite the flu's elusive nature, these predictions have been remarkably accurate in recent years. Even when the virus mutates after the vaccine is developed, the vaccination often provides enough protection to reduce the severity and duration of the illness. Moreover, widespread vaccination contributes to herd immunity, protecting those who cannot be vaccinated by reducing the virus's circulation.

The flu shot, containing an inactivated virus, cannot cause the flu. Some regions use an inhaled vaccine with a weakened live virus, safe for most but not for those with compromised immune systems. Meanwhile, the scientific community is working towards a universal flu vaccine, one that could protect against all strains,

even mutated ones.

Until that breakthrough, the annual hunt for the next year's flu vaccine continues, a testament to human resilience and ingenuity in the face of a constantly evolving viral foe.

# Milk: A Tale of Nourishment and Innovation

In the grand narrative of human consumption, milk holds a special place. It's not just a drink; it's a symbol of life's beginning, a primary source of nourishment that has evolved alongside humanity. But why do humans consume so much milk, and why do we have preferences for certain types over others?

Milk's story begins at birth. It's the first substance we consume, a complete nutritional package perfectly designed for newborns. Containing proteins, carbohydrates, fats, vitamins, minerals, and water, milk is all a baby needs for the first six months of life. This liquid gold's composition varies across species, influenced by factors like diet and environment. For instance, the reindeer of the Arctic Circle produce a milk that's about 20% fat to help their young survive in freezing temperatures.

The process of milk production is a marvel of nature. In mammals, a special class of cells known as mammocytes synthesizes milk. These cells absorb nutrients and synthesize fat droplets, which combine with other molecules and are stored in spaces between cells. The milk is then secreted through various mammalian adaptations, from breasts to udders, and even, in the case of the platypus, through abdominal ducts.

Interestingly, milk production isn't exclusive to females in some species, with instances of lactating males in fruit bats, goats, and cats. Humans have harnessed milk from a variety of animals, including buffalo, goats, sheep, camels, yaks, horses, and cows. Cows, in particular, became the primary source due to their ease of domestication and the similarity of their milk to human milk in terms of fat content.

The dairy industry has transformed milk production from a natural, on-demand process to a large-scale operation to meet consumer demand. Techniques like centrifugation separate milk into cream and liquid, allowing for the creation of diverse dairy products. The fat content of milk is carefully controlled, with full-fat, low-fat, and skim options catering to different preferences.

Homogenization and heat treatments like pasteurization and ultra-high temperature processing ensure milk's safety and extend its shelf life. While these processes are essential for eliminating harmful microbes, they have sparked debates about their impact on milk's nutritional value.

Milk's journey from a simple, essential nutrient to a diverse and widely consumed commodity reflects both human ingenuity and our changing dietary needs. With over 840 million tons of dairy products produced annually, milk's story is one of adaptation, innovation, and enduring significance in our diets.

## The Weight of the World: A Journey from Survival to Epidemic

In the annals of human history, body fat has played a pivotal role, a silent guardian and a reservoir of sustenance, ensuring survival through the harshest of times. This tale of evolution and adaptation begins in the prehistoric era, where natural selection favored those who could store the most fat, a vital trait in an age where chronic malnutrition was the norm.

As the pages of time turned, the narrative of body fat took a dramatic shift. It wasn't until the 18th century that the medical world began to note the negative impacts of being overweight. This change coincided with technological advancements and public health measures that significantly improved the quantity, quality, and variety of food available. An era of abundance dawned, and with it, a healthier population that thrived economically. However, this prosperity came with an unintended consequence – an increase in leisure time and, subsequently, waistlines.

By the mid-19th century, the concept of obesity emerged, marking a stark contrast from the past. What was once a survival advantage had morphed into a cause of ill health, and by another century, it was declared deadly. The distinction between being overweight and obese was quantified by the Body Mass Index (BMI), a simple calculation that, while useful, required additional
factors like waist circumference and muscle mass for accuracy.
The root of obesity is an energy imbalance – consuming more calories than are expended. This imbalance is often the result of a complex interplay of lifestyle choices, environmental factors, and genetic predispositions. Despite recommendations for regular physical activity, a significant portion of the global population remains inactive. The rise of calorie-dense processed foods, larger portion sizes, and aggressive marketing strategies contribute to passive overeating. Moreover, socio-economic disparities exacerbate the risk, with disadvantaged communities facing greater challenges in accessing healthy, affordable food options.

Genetics, too, play a crucial role in this narrative. Research involving families and separated twins has demonstrated a hereditary link to weight gain. Recent studies have even uncovered connections between obesity and variations in gut bacteria. This multifaceted issue has escalated into a global epidemic, indiscriminately affecting all ages, genders, and socio-economic groups across both developed and developing nations. Alarmingly, child obesity has surged by 60% in just two decades, underscoring the urgency of the situation.

The path to recovery for those with obesity is fraught with challenges. Hormonal and metabolic changes diminish the body's response to overeating, and weight loss efforts are often met with reduced calorie burning compared to individuals who have never been overweight. Additionally, as weight increases, the brain's ability to regulate food intake and fat storage becomes impaired. However, there is hope. Evidence suggests that long-term, well-monitored behavioral changes can lead to improvements in obesity-related health issues, and interventions like bariatric surgery can have significant benefits.

In conclusion, what was once an evolutionary advantage for survival has turned into a formidable adversary in the modern world. As the global population continues to grapple with this epidemic, a concerted effort towards healthier lifestyles and global preventive measures becomes imperative. Obesity is no longer an isolated issue; it is a weight that the world must collectively strive to manage.

# Retinal Regeneration: Lessons from the Zebrafish

Imagine a world where losing your sight isn't irreversible, where the human eye could repair itself like a masterful self-healing machine. This isn't science fiction; it's a possibility scientists are exploring by studying the remarkable zebrafish.

For individuals suffering from diseases like retinitis pigmentosa and Usher's syndrome, vision loss is a grim reality. These conditions progressively damage the retina, the light-sensitive layer at the back of the eye crucial for vision. The human retina, composed of rod and cone photoreceptors, translates light into neural signals, enabling us to see. Unfortunately, in these diseases, the photoreceptors deteriorate, leading to eventual blindness.

The human body, unlike some of its aquatic counterparts, cannot regenerate these vital photoreceptors. We're born with a finite number, which explains why babies have disproportionately large, adorable eyes. But what if we could unlock the secret to regenerating these crucial cells?

Enter the zebrafish, an unassuming yet extraordinary creature capable of regenerating various body parts, including its retina. When zebrafish photoreceptors are damaged, they don't just heal; they regenerate and reconnect to the brain, restoring vision. This remarkable ability has made the zebrafish a subject of intense study, as

its retinal structure closely mirrors that of humans.

Scientists have successfully replicated human retinal disorders in zebrafish, providing a unique window into the regenerative process. The key players in this process are the Müller glia cells. In response to damage, these cells undergo a remarkable transformation, adopting characteristics of stem cells, which can morph into any cell type. These transformed cells then divide, creating new photoreceptors that migrate to the retina and integrate into the neural circuitry.

Recent research has shed light on potential triggers for this transformation. In mice, certain chemicals like glutamate and amino adipate have spurred Müller glia to divide and evolve into photoreceptors. This discovery is akin to finding a secret code that replenishes a dwindling army, offering a glimmer of hope for human application.

However, numerous questions remain. Can we replicate this Müller glia transformation in the human eye? What controls this process, and how do the new photoreceptors seamlessly integrate into the existing retinal structure? Is this regenerative capability a lost trait in humans, or does it lie dormant, waiting to be awakened?

The path to applying these findings to human medicine is fraught with complexity. The evolutionary divergence between humans and zebrafish means that what works in one may not directly translate to the other. Yet, the potential is too great to ignore. Understanding and harnessing this regenerative power could revolutionize the treatment of blindness and vision impairment.

As research progresses, the zebrafish continues to be a beacon of hope, a tiny creature with a monumental lesson to teach. The quest to unlock the secrets of retinal regeneration is not just about restoring sight; it's about redefining the limits of human healing and resilience.

## The Fiery Dance: Unraveling the Mystery of Spiciness

Why does a bite of a spicy pepper send waves of fire through your mouth? What mysterious alchemy makes wasabi a tear-inducing experience? And just how spicy can spices get? To understand this culinary conundrum, we must delve into the essence of spiciness.

Spiciness, contrary to common belief, is not a taste like sweetness or sourness. It's a sensation, a complex interaction between certain food compounds and our sensory neurons. Specifically, it involves polymodal nociceptors, sensory neurons that are scattered throughout our body, including in our mouth and nose. These receptors are also activated by extreme heat, which is why consuming a chili pepper can feel akin to touching a hot stove.

Interestingly, when you eat something containing menthol, such as mint, it triggers a completely different sensation. The cool, minty compound activates your cold receptors, offering a refreshing contrast to the heat of spiciness.

When these heat-sensitive receptors are activated by spicy foods, your body reacts as if it's in contact with a high-temperature source. This explains the sweating and the quickened heartbeat, a fight-or-flight response akin to reacting to a threat.

Not all spicy experiences are created equal, though. The difference lies in the specific compounds involved. Capsaicin in chili peppers and piperine in black pepper are larger molecules that primarily affect the mouth. In contrast, mustard, horseradish, and wasabi contain smaller molecules that rise into the sinuses, explaining why wasabi hits your nasal passages hard.

The spiciness of food is quantified using the Scoville scale, which measures the dilution required for the heat of capsaicin to become undetectable. For perspective, a sweet bell pepper scores zero on this scale, while Tabasco sauce ranges between 1,200 and 1,400 Scoville units. The real heavyweights, like the Trinidad Moruga Scorpion and the Carolina Reaper, register between 1.5 and 2 million units, nearing the intensity of pepper spray.

The human fascination with spicy food is an enigma. Archaeological evidence suggests that our ancestors used spices as far back as 23,000 years ago, but the reasons remain unclear. Were these spices used for culinary, medicinal, or purely decorative purposes? More recent findings, like a 6,000-year-old pot with traces of mustard, hint at culinary uses.

One theory posits that spices were initially used to combat foodborne bacteria, particularly in warmer climates where such microbes thrive. Today, the allure of spicy food might be akin to the thrill of a roller coaster – a love for the adrenaline rush despite the immediate discomfort.

Interestingly, a penchant for spicy food might be ingrained in our genes. And for those who aspire to increase their spice tolerance, be warned: studies suggest that the pain doesn't diminish with exposure. Instead, you might just become more accepting, even appreciative, of the fiery sensation.

So, as you venture into the world of spicy cuisine, remember that it's not just about challenging your taste buds. It's about embracing a complex interplay of biology, history, and personal preference. In the realm of spicy foods, the burn is inevitable, but the journey is uniquely exhilarating.

## The Rhythms of Red: Understanding the Menstrual Cycle

In a world teeming with diverse life, there exists a universal experience shared by approximately 300 million women at any given moment: menstruation. This monthly cycle, a dance of hormones and biology, is a profound rhythm shared by women worldwide.

The menstrual cycle, a 28-day rotation marked by a period lasting between two and seven days, is a marvel of the human body's complexity. This cycle, repeating roughly 450 times during a woman's life, is orchestrated by a symphony of hormonal controls, fine-tuning the body's internal workings.

At the heart of this process are the ovaries, each a tiny universe of follicles containing oocytes, or unfertilized egg cells. From the onset of puberty, these ovaries embark on a remarkable journey, releasing one egg each month, either culminating in pregnancy or a period.

The cycle begins with the pituitary gland, a hormone maestro in the brain, releasing follicle-stimulating hormone (FSH) and luteinizing hormone (LH) into the bloodstream. These hormones travel to the ovaries, prompting the egg cells to mature, while the follicles produce estrogen. This hormonal interplay is a delicate balance, with estrogen peaking and then signaling the pituitary to release more LH, leading to ovulation.

Ovulation, the release of the most mature egg

from the ovary, is a pivotal moment in the cycle, occurring typically 10 to 16 days before the period begins. The oocyte's journey through the fallopian tube is brief, with a narrow window for fertilization. If unfertilized, the egg's journey ends, closing the opportunity for pregnancy that month.

Post-ovulation, the empty follicle transforms, secreting progesterone, preparing the womb's lining for a potential pregnancy. If no fertilized egg embeds, estrogen and progesterone levels drop, the womb lining degenerates, and the period begins, shedding blood and tissue.

This cycle is not just a biological process but a narrative of potential life. Each month is a story of preparation and transformation, with the womb readying itself for a possible new beginning or resetting for the next opportunity.

Yet, this seemingly clockwork cycle is as unique as the individuals it affects. Variations in timing, duration, and experience of menstrual cycles are normal, reflecting the diversity of women's bodies. These differences underscore the importance of understanding and embracing this natural process.

Understanding menstruation is empowering. It offers women insight into their bodies, enabling them to navigate and harmonize with this intricate cycle. This knowledge is not just about managing a biological function but about connecting with a fundamental aspect of womanhood.

In a world where every day is a blend of shared experiences and individual stories, menstruation is a powerful reminder of the common threads that bind us and the unique rhythms that define us. It's a cycle not just of biology but of life itself, a rhythm that resonates with the heartbeat of womanhood.

## Why should we use sunscreen?

The sun: a celestial giant that warms our planet, nurtures our crops, and brightens our days. Yet, this same life-giving star can be a subtle adversary, casting ultraviolet rays that threaten our skin's health. This is the story of sunscreen, our shield against the sun's darker side.

Sunscreen is more than just a summer accessory; it's a crucial defender in our daily health regimen. It's the invisible armor designed to protect us from sunburn, premature aging, and the insidious threat of skin cancer. But how does this unassuming lotion achieve such a feat?

The sun bombards us with different types of ultraviolet rays, primarily UVA and UVB. Each type affects our skin differently, from accelerating aging to increasing our risk of skin cancer. The key players in our skin's reaction to these rays are melanin, the pigment that colors our skin, and hemoglobin, found in our red blood cells.

Enter sunscreen, with its two main types: physical and chemical blockers. Physical blockers, like zinc oxide and titanium dioxide, act as a literal shield, reflecting the sun's rays. These are the sunscreens that leave a visible trace, a reminder of their protective presence.

Chemical blockers, on the other hand, absorb these rays. They're often more user-friendly, blending invisibly into the skin, but they can deteriorate more quickly under the sun's assault. Each type of sunscreen undergoes rigorous testing to determine its Sunburn Protection Factor (SPF), a measure of how well it guards against UVB rays.

But sunscreen isn't just for those prone to sunburn. Its protective embrace is essential for all, regardless of skin tone. Even those who don't burn easily need defense against UVA rays. And for the very young, whose skin is especially vulnerable, sunscreen is a critical shield.

The stakes are high. Every day, the DNA in our skin cells battles against mutations, many caused by the sun's ultraviolet rays. These mutations can lead to uncontrolled cell growth – the hallmark of skin cancer. And while the threat is invisible, its effects can be devastating.

Beyond health, there's also the matter of aesthetics. Sun damage is a leading cause of premature aging. Chronic exposure to the sun can rob the skin of its elasticity, leading to a saggy, weathered appearance. This isn't just speculation; it's visibly evident in those who've had prolonged sun exposure on one side of their face, like truck drivers.

So, how do we best use this essential tool? Apply sunscreen generously and regularly, especially during prolonged exposure or in environments where the sun's rays are amplified. But don't just rely on sunscreen alone. Protective clothing, shade, and avoiding the sun during its peak hours are all part of a comprehensive sun protection strategy.

When choosing a sunscreen, look for broad-spectrum coverage, an SPF of at least 30, and water resistance. And remember, sprays may be convenient, but they require a generous and thorough application.

In the end, sunscreen is more than just a lotion; it's a testament to our understanding of the sun's dual nature. It allows us to embrace the warmth and beauty of the sun while respecting its power. So, as you step out into the sunlight, remember to arm yourself with sunscreen – your faithful guardian against the hidden perils of our brightest star.

## The Art of Alignment: Mastering Posture in a Slouching World

"Stand up straight!" How often have you heard that nagging reminder? It might seem like just another old adage, but the truth is, your posture – the way you hold your body when you're sitting or standing – is the cornerstone of your physical well-being. It's the unsung hero in the story of how your body copes with the relentless tug of gravity and the myriad stresses of daily life.

In a world increasingly dominated by screens and sedentary lifestyles, maintaining good posture is becoming a lost art. Yet, it's more crucial than ever. When your posture is off-kilter, it's not just about not looking your best. It's about an internal battle where muscles strain, joints creak, and your body labors tirelessly to keep you upright and balanced.

Imagine your body as a finely tuned structure, a skyscraper of bones and muscles. When everything is aligned – when the 33 vertebrae of your spine stack up just right – your body moves with grace and efficiency. But when things are out of whack, it's like a building starting to lean, straining under its own weight.

This story isn't just about bones and muscles, though. It's about how poor posture can be a silent saboteur, contributing to a range of woes from tension headaches to back pain. It's about how the way you carry yourself can even echo in your emotional state and your perception of pain.

But here's the twist: achieving good posture isn't as straightforward as it once was. Our modern lifestyle, with its awkward sitting positions and downward gazes at devices, is reshaping our bodies. Studies are sounding the alarm – our collective posture is on the decline.

So, what's the blueprint for good posture? Picture the spine not as a rigid rod but as an elegant S-curve, a shock absorber that distributes the stress of movement. When standing, imagine a plumb line running from just in front of your knee to a few inches in front of your ankle – that's the sweet spot of balance. Sitting? Think right angles at your knees, a straight neck, relaxed shoulders, and feet firmly planted on the ground.

If your posture is less than ideal, don't despair. The path to better posture isn't paved with just reminders to sit up straight. It's about redesigning your environment – from the height of your screen to the way you sleep. It's about choosing shoes that support your arches and using headsets to avoid cradling the phone.

But here's the key: good posture isn't a static state. It's about movement, about keeping the body fluid and dynamic. Even perfect posture can't make up for the perils of staying still for too long. Regular movement, smart lifting, and balanced exercise – these are the true heroes in the quest for better posture.

In the end, this story isn't just about standing up straight. It's a tale of how, in a world that often encourages us to slouch, both physically and metaphorically, maintaining good posture is a quiet act of rebellion. It's a commitment to holding yourself in a way that respects the intricate architecture of your body. So, the next time you hear "Stand up straight," remember, it's not just a command – it's an invitation to a healthier, more aligned life.

# A Journey Through the Kidneys' Marvelous World

On a scorching summer day, you find relief in gulping down several glasses of water, one after the other. But what follows next is a fascinating tale of biology, a story of two bean-shaped heroes residing within you, performing a balancing act so intricate it could rival any high-wire circus act. These are your kidneys, the unsung guardians of your body's internal equilibrium.

Imagine this: every day, your body's entire blood supply circulates through these two remarkable organs many times. This means that in just 24 hours, your kidneys filter around 180 liters of blood. It's a relentless job, necessitated by the constant changes in your blood's composition as you consume food and drink.

Blood enters each kidney through a maze of arteries that keep branching out into tinier vessels. These vessels intertwine with a million nephrons in each kidney, forming a sophisticated network of filters and sensors. It's here, in these nephrons, that the magic of filtration and fine-tuning occurs.

Each nephron is equipped with a glomerulus and a tubule – the former acting like a sieve, allowing only specific ingredients like vitamins and minerals to pass through, while the latter plays detective, deciding what the body needs to reabsorb and what it needs to discard.

But it's not just about filtering the good from the bad. The kidneys are also masterful waste managers. They identify unwanted elements like urea, a byproduct of protein breakdown, and efficiently convert them into urine. This urine then travels through the ureters, two long channels, finally reaching the bladder for disposal.

And then there's the matter of water – the essence of life. Drink too much, and your kidneys swiftly work to balance your body's fluid levels by sending the excess to the bladder. Drink too little, and they cleverly conserve water, sending only a minimal amount to the bladder, which explains why your urine gets darker when you're dehydrated.

But the kidneys' talents extend beyond filtration and fluid balance. They are biochemical alchemists, activating vitamin D, secreting renin to regulate blood pressure, and producing erythropoietin to boost red blood cell production. Without these functions, our bodies would be in a state of constant disarray, overwhelmed by the buildup of waste and unregulated fluid levels.

So, the next time you feel the urge to visit the restroom after quenching your thirst, remember the incredible journey that's taking place within you. It's a journey of two magical beans – your kidneys – tirelessly working not just to maintain a delicate balance, but to sustain life itself.

## The Hangover Experiment: A Spirited Journey Through Science and Spirits

In 1973, a unique experiment unfolded, one that would resonate with anyone who's ever woken up with a pounding headache and a vow never to drink again. Twenty volunteers embarked on an eight-week journey, not of self-discovery, but of scientific inquiry – getting systematically inebriated on a variety of alcoholic beverages. Their mission? To determine which drinks were the worst culprits for hangovers.

This study, though small, was a stepping stone in understanding the enigmatic hangover. At its core, ethanol – the molecule we commonly refer to as alcohol – was identified as the primary instigator. Present in all alcoholic drinks, its quantity largely dictates the hangover's intensity. Yet, individual experiences vary, influenced by factors like weight, age, genetics, and more.

Hangovers, despite their varied symptoms, share a common thread of discomfort. But what exactly happens in our bodies during a hangover? Alcohol, it turns out, is a master of disruption, meddling with neural communication and throwing the brain into a hyperactive state as alcohol levels drop. This leads to the tremors, rapid heartbeat, and restless sleep that many experience.

The plot thickens as we delve deeper into alcohol's effects. It disrupts hormonal balances, including cortisol, which regulates wakefulness, and vasopressin, which controls urine production. The result? Dehydration, leading to the classic hangover symptoms of thirst, dry mouth, and the dreaded headache.

But there's more. Alcohol's influence extends to neurotransmitters involved in pain signaling, mitochondria responsible for energy production, and even the immune system, causing inflammation that can affect mood and memory. It irritates the gastrointestinal tract, leading to stomach pain, nausea, and vomiting.

Interestingly, the type of alcoholic beverage plays a role too. Methanol, a byproduct of fermentation found in certain drinks, is particularly notorious for exacerbating hangover symptoms. Beverages closer to pure ethanol, like gin and vodka, tend to be less punishing, while those rich in flavor compounds, such as whiskey, brandy, and red wine, might pack a heavier hangover punch.

So, what about the myriad hangover remedies touted over the years? Hydration with water and electrolytes can alleviate dehydration-related symptoms, and carbs can help restore depleted glucose levels. Yet, the only foolproof method to avoid a hangover remains moderation or abstinence.

This story, spanning from the first alcoholic beverages consumed around 7000 BCE to modern scientific studies, is not just about hangovers. It's a tale of human curiosity, the pursuit of understanding our body's reactions to alcohol, and the quest for that elusive, perfect remedy for the morning after. In this spirited journey through science and spirits, one truth remains clear: when it comes to alcohol, the choices we make have consequences, some more lasting than others.

## The Bald Truth: A Tale of Hair, Science, and Self-Acceptance

What do Jeff Bezos, Yoda, and The Rock have in common? They, like many other historical and fictive individuals, are bald, in some cases by their own choice. For centuries, a shining dome has been a symbol of intelligence, but despite this, many balding people still wish their hair would return. This smooth scalp, often seen as a mark of wisdom, has been a subject of both admiration and consternation. For many who watch their hairlines recede, the question looms: Why does hair loss occur, and can science reverse this seemingly relentless tide?

The story begins with a look at the average human head, a bustling metropolis of 100,000 to 150,000 hair strands. Scientists, in their quest to understand this complex ecosystem, have unearthed two key insights. Firstly, the visible hair is largely composed of keratin, a protein that remains after cells die and are pushed upwards by new growth. Secondly, the real heroes of hair growth are the hair follicles, intricate organs that form pre-birth and cycle through growth phases throughout our lives.

This cycle comprises three phases. The first, anagen, is the growth stage where the majority of follicles are actively pushing hair at about 1 centimeter per month. This phase can last from two to seven years, influenced heavily by genetics. Following this is catagen, a regressive stage where follicles shrink and cut off blood supply, preparing the hair to be shed. This lasts a mere two to three weeks. Finally, there's telogen, a resting phase lasting about 10 to 12 weeks, during which hair shedding is normal and expected.

However, not all follicles follow this script. In male pattern baldness, which accounts for 95% of men's baldness, follicles become hypersensitive to dihydrotestosterone (DHT), a derivative of testosterone. This sensitivity leads to follicle shrinkage, resulting in hair that's thinner and more fragile. The progression of this baldness follows the Norwood Scale, a measure of severity that starts with receding hairlines and culminates in a sparse ring of hair.

But genetics isn't the sole culprit in hair loss. Stress, for instance, can shock follicles into premature resting phases. Women often experience this post-childbirth. Additionally, certain conditions and treatments, like chemotherapy, can disrupt the growth phase, anagen.

Yet, there's a glimmer of hope in this tale of loss. Scientific exploration has revealed that the roots of hair often remain alive beneath the skin's surface. Armed with this knowledge, researchers have developed treatments that shorten the resting phase and kickstart the growth phase. Other treatments target male pattern baldness by inhibiting the conversion of testosterone to DHT. The frontier of this scientific saga is the exploration of stem cells, which regulate the hair growth cycle. Scientists are investigating ways to manipulate these cells to rejuvenate dormant follicles.

As this story of hair loss and scientific endeavor unfolds, those experiencing baldness can take solace in the fact that they share this journey with some of the most remarkable figures in history and fiction. In the quest for hair revival, science marches on, but in the meantime, the state of being bald remains a symbol of distinction, a testament to the diverse tapestry of human appearance.

## Bloodlines: The Genetic Story of A, B, AB, and O

In the grand tapestry of human existence, a common thread binds us all: the blood that courses through our veins. Yet, this seemingly universal lifeline is more complex and varied than one might initially believe. This story begins with a journey into the microscopic world of our blood, a world where the drama of survival and the mysteries of genetics play out every moment. At the center of this narrative are red blood cells, the diligent couriers of oxygen, thanks to a protein called hemoglobin. But these cells harbor another, more discreet element on their outer membrane - proteins known as antigens. These are not just mere components; they are the critical communicators with white blood cells, the vigilant guardians of our immune system. Antigens are like the secret handshakes of the cellular world, telling the immune system to recognize these cells as part of the body, not as foreign invaders.

The plot thickens with the introduction of two main types of these antigens, A and B, the key players in determining your blood type. But how do we arrive at four primary blood types from only two antigens? The answer lies in the genetic script of our being, written in alleles - A, B, and O. The A and B alleles are like the dominant characters in this genetic story, coding for their respective antigens. In contrast, the O allele is the understudy, coding for neither antigen.

Every person inherits a pair of these alleles, one from each parent, which combine to determine their blood type. The A and B alleles, both dominant, can either team up or stand alone, creating types A, B, or AB. The O allele, being recessive, only makes its presence known when paired with another O, leading to type O blood.

This genetic interplay is not just a matter of identity; it's a critical factor in life-saving medical procedures like blood transfusions. If someone with type A blood receives type B, their body's defense system springs into action, attacking the foreign antigens and potentially causing a dangerous reaction. But those with type AB blood are like the diplomats of this cellular world, accepting both A and B antigens without conflict, making them universal recipients.

Conversely, individuals with type O blood are the altruistic donors, their blood compatible with any recipient. However, they must be cautious, as their immune system will not tolerate any blood type other than their own.

Yet, this genetic drama is further complicated by another character: the Rh factor. Discovered in rhesus monkeys, this factor adds another layer to the blood type puzzle, denoted as Rh positive or Rh negative. It plays a crucial role not only in transfusions but also in the narrative of pregnancy. An Rh negative mother carrying an Rh positive child can face a perilous situation, as her body may produce antibodies that attack the fetus, leading to hemolytic disease of the newborn.

While some cultures weave tales linking blood type to personality, science paints a different picture. The reasons behind the evolution of blood types remain a mystery, perhaps a defense against diseases or a product of genetic drift.

In the end, the story of blood types is a fascinating journey through genetics, immunology, and medicine. It's a reminder of our shared humanity, yet a testament to our incredible diversity, a complexity hidden within the very essence of life that flows within us all.

## Why is meningitis so dangerous?

In the sweltering heat of 1987, Saudi Arabia was teeming with life as tens of thousands of pilgrims converged for the annual Hajj. A journey of faith and devotion soon turned into a medical nightmare. Within days of the pilgrimage's conclusion, a menacing shadow loomed over the joyous gathering. More than 2,000 cases of meningitis erupted, not just within Saudi Arabia, but spiraling across the globe.

Meningitis, the inflammation of the protective membranes covering the brain and spinal cord, is a formidable adversary in the realm of infectious diseases. Its notoriety stems from its rapid onslaught; in severe cases, it can claim a life in less than 24 hours. Yet, with prompt medical intervention, the grim reaper's grasp can often be evaded.

The disease manifests in three primary forms: fungal, viral, and bacterial, with the latter being the most lethal. Bacterial meningitis is a master of stealth and speed. It infiltrates the human body through airborne droplets from an infected person's sneeze or cough. It can also spread through intimate acts like kissing or sharing personal items.

Carriers of the bacteria can be asymptomatic, unwittingly becoming agents of its rapid dissemination. Once the bacteria breach the defenses of the nose, mouth, and throat, they embark on a sinister journey through the bloodstream, heading straight for the brain.

The blood-brain barrier, a fortress of tightly packed cells guarding the brain, usually blocks unauthorized entry. However, meningitis bacteria possess a cunning ability to deceive this barrier, gaining entry into the brain. Once inside, they launch an assault on the meninges, triggering a fierce inflammatory response. The symptoms are brutal: fever, debilitating headaches, and a neck so stiff it feels like iron.

As the bacteria proliferate, they unleash toxins that lead to septicemia, or blood poisoning. This causes blood vessels to break down, resulting in a rash that soon morphs into large, sinister blotches under the skin. These toxins also deplete oxygen in the blood, jeopardizing vital organs and increasing the risk of organ failure and death.

Despite its ferocity, meningitis is not a death sentence. Modern medicine has honed its ability to combat this disease, significantly lowering mortality rates with timely treatment. However, delay in seeking medical help can have dire consequences, including the risk of amputation due to cell death in extremities, or even long-term brain damage and memory loss.

Prevention, as always, is better than cure. Vaccines against the deadliest strains of meningitis are a shield for those most vulnerable: young children, the immunocompromised, and those in large gatherings where an outbreak could wreak havoc.

Meningitis is a global concern, with a notorious prevalence in the 'meningitis belt' stretching across Africa. Yet, it does not discriminate by geography. If meningitis symptoms arise, immediate medical attention is crucial.

The 1987 Hajj outbreak serves as a stark reminder of meningitis's potential wrath. It underscores the importance of vigilance, rapid response, and the power of vaccines in our ongoing battle against this invisible enemy.

## The Shape of Nutrition: Olive Oil vs. Pancake Mix, the fat we eat.

In a world where the word 'fat' often sends shivers down the spines of health-conscious individuals, a surprising truth lurks beneath the surface of our everyday foods. Picture this: a bottle of pure, glistening olive oil, and beside it, a box of pancake mix. At first glance, one might hastily label the oil as the dietary villain, being 100% fat, while the pancake mix, with a modest 11% fat content, seems like a safer bet. But here's the twist – the olive oil is actually the hero of this story, and the pancake mix? Not so much. The journey to understanding this paradox begins with a simple question: What is fat? Let's dive into the microscopic world of a salmon, a creature celebrated for its healthy fats. Zooming past organs and tissues, down to the cellular level, we encounter molecules called triglycerides. These are the building blocks of fat, but they're far from uniform.

Imagine a molecule with a backbone – that's glycerol, the anchor of our story. Attached to it are three chains, known as fatty acids. It's the structure of these chains that dictates whether a fat is a friend or foe to our health. Some fatty acids are short, others long. But the real game-changer is the type of bonds linking the carbon atoms in these chains.

There are two main characters in our fatty acid tale: saturated and unsaturated fats. Saturated fats, laden with single bonds, are often the villains, especially when consumed in excess. Unsaturated fats, featuring at least one double bond, are usually the protagonists. But even among these, there's a plot twist.

Double bonds in unsaturated fats can be arranged in two ways, creating entirely different substances. The first arrangement, called 'cis', is relatively unknown. The second, 'trans', is infamous. Trans fats, despite being unsaturated, are like undercover antagonists, wreaking havoc on our health. They're stable, they don't spoil easily, and they're great for cooking, but their impact on our body is nefariously profound.

The reason? It all boils down to shape. In the intricate world of biochemistry, shape dictates function. The 3D structure of a molecule determines where it fits, where it doesn't, and what processes it disrupts in our body. Trans fats, with their unique shape, interfere in ways that are far more harmful than any other type of fat.

So, how do we spot these culprits in our food? The secret lies in the words 'partially hydrogenated' on ingredient lists. Despite what nutrition labels claim, if you see these words, trans fats are lurking there. The FDA's labeling laws have loopholes, allowing foods with less than half a gram of trans fat per serving to claim they have none. But the size of a 'serving' can be misleadingly small.

Returning to our olive oil and pancake mix, the truth becomes clear. Olive oil, rich in unsaturated fats and free from trans fats, is a champion for our

health. The pancake mix, however, hides its villains – saturated and trans fats – behind a facade of low overall fat content.

This tale isn't just about olive oil and pancake mix. It's a broader narrative about the types of fat we consume. The moral? It's not the quantity of fat that matters most, but its quality and shape. In the complex dance of molecules within our bodies, shape is everything, and understanding this can transform our approach to what we eat.

## The Birth of Vaccination

In the spring of 1796, in a small English village, a daring experiment was about to unfold, one that would pivot the course of medical history. Edward Jenner, a scientist with a revolutionary hunch, stood ready to test a theory that seemed as wild as it was hopeful. His subject? An eight-year-old boy, his tool? A virus, drawn not from a human, but a cow.

Jenner's hypothesis was simple yet groundbreaking. He believed that cowpox, a disease common in cattle but mild in humans, could offer protection against the deadly smallpox virus. The world around him was ravaged by smallpox outbreaks, each wave leaving death and despair in its wake. Jenner's solution, if successful, promised a shield against this invisible enemy.

The boy, young and unaware of the significance of the moment, watched as Jenner injected him with material from a cowpox blister. It was a gamble, a leap into the unknown. Days passed, and the village held its breath. Then, something remarkable happened – or rather, didn't happen. The boy remained healthy, unscathed by smallpox. Jenner's theory had not only held but triumphed. This was the birth of the first-ever vaccine.

But why did Jenner's experiment work? To grasp this, we must dive into the intricate world of the human immune system. When we encounter harmful microbes, our bodies launch a defense, marked by coughs, sneezes, fever – all signs of our immune system at war. This is just the first wave of defense, known as innate immunity.

The real game-changer, however, lies in our second line of defense: adaptive immunity. This involves special cells – B-cells and T-cells – that not only fight off invaders but remember them. It's like having a personal army that not only defeats the enemy but keeps a detailed record of their tactics for future battles.

However, this incredible system has its limits. It needs time to learn and adapt, and sometimes, time is a luxury we don't have, especially when faced with a formidable foe like smallpox. This is where Jenner's genius shone. What if we could 'train' our immune system in advance, prepare it for battle before the enemy even strikes?

Vaccines do just that. They mimic an infection, triggering our adaptive immune system without subjecting us to the disease's full brutality. Over time, scientists have developed various types of vaccines. Live attenuated vaccines use a weakened form of the virus, while inactivated vaccines contain killed pathogens. Both teach the body to recognize and combat the invaders without causing the actual disease.

But these methods have their drawbacks. Live vaccines can be too robust for those with weaker immune systems, and inactivated ones may not offer long-lasting immunity. Enter subunit vaccines, which use only a part of the pathogen, focusing the immune response more precisely.

The frontier of vaccine science is even more exciting. DNA vaccines, a novel approach, use specific genes from a pathogen to trigger an immune response. Injected into the body, these genes instruct our cells to produce antigens, priming our immune system against future attacks. This method holds immense promise, potentially offering more effective defenses against elusive enemies like HIV, malaria, or Ebola.

Edward Jenner's leap into the unknown laid the foundation for this journey. His cowpox experiment, a moment of audacious hope, has spiraled into a saga of scientific triumph. From that small English village to labs across the world, the quest continues, each breakthrough a testament to the enduring power of human curiosity and the relentless pursuit of a healthier, safer world.

## A Journey Through Memory Lane: Why Some Memories Fade Away?

Let's dive into the mysterious world of memories, where some moments stay etched in our minds while others slip through the cracks of time. Ever wonder why we remember that vivid childhood memory so well, but can't recall what we had for lunch three weeks ago? It's a memory puzzle worth solving.

Picture this: you're dialing a phone number. The experience transforms into a surge of electrical energy racing along a network of neurons. Initially, it lands in your short-term memory, a temporary storage spot lasting from a few seconds to a couple of minutes. From there, it's shuttled to long-term memory, with key players like the hippocampus making it all happen. Finally, these memories find their cozy homes in various brain regions.

Now, here's where it gets fascinating. Neurons across your brain chat through tiny junctions called synapses, using specialized messengers called neurotransmitters. If two neurons engage in frequent conversations, something magical unfolds. Their communication becomes more efficient, a phenomenon known as "long-term potentiation." This, my friends, is the secret sauce behind storing long-term memories.

But why do some memories pull a vanishing act? Well, age is one factor to consider. As the years roll on, synapses can start to misbehave, weakening the retrieval of memories. Scientists propose several theories, from the shrinking of our brains (the hippocampus loses 5% of neurons per decade, totaling 20% by age 80) to dwindling neurotransmitter production, like acetylcholine, a memory maestro.

Remember that memories are etched most vividly when we're focused, engaged, and find meaning in the information. Sadly, aging comes with its baggage. Mental and physical health issues that often accompany the golden years can mess with our attention, making memories slip through our fingers.

Enter chronic stress, a notorious memory thief. When stress is a constant companion, our bodies go into hyper-alert mode. While this is an evolutionary defense mechanism, it has downsides. The excess stress chemicals can damage brain cells and hinder new ones from forming, ultimately affecting our memory retention.

Depression is another antagonist in the memory tale. Those grappling with depression are 40% more likely to face memory woes. Low serotonin levels, linked to alertness, can make it challenging to stay attentive to new info. Dwelling on past sorrows, a common trait in depression, can further divert our attention from the present, impairing short-term memory.

And let's not forget isolation, a close friend of depression. Studies from the Harvard School of Public Health hint that folks with robust social ties

experience slower memory decline as they age. While the exact mechanism remains a bit mysterious, experts suspect that social interactions give our brains a much-needed mental workout. Just like your muscles, you've got to use your brain, or it might just decide to take a snooze.

But fear not, dear reader, for there are steps you can take to help your brain preserve those precious memories. Keep that body in motion to boost blood flow to the brain. Nourish yourself with a balanced diet to provide your brain with the essential nutrients it craves. And last but not least, give your brain a good workout. Challenge it with new experiences, like learning a new language—it's one of the best defenses against memory loss.

So, the next time a memory slips away like a whisper in the wind, remember that your brain is a complex labyrinth, and sometimes, even the most vivid moments can get lost in its twists and turns. But with some mental gymnastics, you can keep those memories alive and thriving.

## Why do we like to be scared?

Gather 'round, brave souls, for we're about to embark on a spine-tingling journey into the enigmatic world of fear. You see, fear is a curious beast—it can both terrify and delight in the same breath. Picture this: people willingly lining up to scare themselves, whether through hair-raising thrill rides or spine-chilling horror movies. It may sound perplexing, but the allure of fear is more than meets the eye.

Fear has a bad rap, but it's not all bad. For starters, fear can actually feel pretty good. When a threat triggers our fight -or -flight response, our bodies prepare for danger by releasing chemicals that change how our brains and bodies function.

This automatic response jump -start systems that can aid in survival. They do this by making sure we have enough energy and are protected from feeling pain, while shutting down non -essential systems, like critical thought.

Feeling pain -free and energized while not getting caught up in worrisome thoughts that normally occupy our brains, that all sounds great. And it can be, because this response is similar, though not exactly the same, to what we experience in positive, high -arousal states, like excitement, happiness, and even during sex.

The difference lays in the context. If we're in real danger, we're focused on survival, not fun. But when we trigger this high -arousal response in a safe place, we can switch over to enjoying the natural high of being scared.

It's why people on roller coasters can go from screaming to laughing within moments. Your body is already in a euphoric state; you're just relabeling the experience. And though the threat response is universal, research shows differences between individuals in how the chemicals associated with the threat are.

threat response work. This explains why some are more prone to thrill -seeking than others. Other normal physical differences explain why some may love the dizziness associated with a loop -the -loop while loathing the stomach drop sensation of a steep roller coaster, or why some squeal with delight inside a haunted house but retreat in terror if taken to an actual cemetery.

Fear brings more than just a fun natural high. Doing things that we're afraid of can give us a nice boost of self -esteem. Like any personal challenge, whether it's running a race or finishing a long book, when we make it through to the end, we feel a sense of accomplishment.

This is true even if we know we're not really in any danger. Our thinking brains may know the zombies aren't real, but our bodies tell us otherwise. The fear feels real, so when we make it through alive, the satisfaction and sense of accomplishment also feel real.

This is a great evolutionary adaptation. Those who had the right balance of bravery and wit to know when to push through the fear and when to retreat were rewarded with survival, new food, and new lands.

Finally, fear can bring people together. Emotions can be contagious, and when you see your friend scream and laugh, you feel compelled to do the same. This is because we make sense of what our friends are experiencing by recreating the experience ourselves.

In fact, the parts of the brain that are active when our friend screams are active in us when we watch them. This not only intensifies our own emotional experience but makes us feel closer to those we're with.

The feeling of closeness during times of fear is aided by the hormone oxytocin, released during fight or flight. Fear is a powerful emotional experience, and anything that triggers a strong reaction is going to be stored in our memory well. You don't want to forget what can hurt you. So, if your memory of watching a horror film with your friends is positive and leaves you with a sense of satisfaction, then you'll want to do it over and over again.

**The risk of mixing drugs.**

In the world of medicine, there's a secret danger that lurks in the shadows, a danger that often goes unnoticed until it strikes. It's called a drug interaction, and it's like a silent saboteur that can wreak havoc on your health. Today, I'm going to take you on a journey into this mysterious realm, where seemingly innocent substances can turn into harmful adversaries.

Imagine three people, each going about their day, unaware of the hidden risks they're taking. One person decides to wash down their cholesterol medication with a glass of grapefruit juice, another takes acetaminophen for a sore ankle just before a night out with friends, and the third, who's already on blood-thinning medication, reaches for an aspirin to quell a nagging headache.

Seems harmless, right? Well, here's the twist – all three of them have unwittingly set the stage for a risky drug interaction, a potentially perilous encounter that could lead to kidney failure, liver damage, or even internal bleeding.

But what exactly are drug interactions, and how do they sneak into our lives? These interactions occur when a drug collides with another substance, creating effects that neither would have on their own. It's like a chemical dance where partners mix, match, and sometimes clash in unexpected ways. These partners can include foods, herbal supplements, legal drugs, and even illicit substances, making it a diverse and unpredictable arena.

Let's break it down further. Drug interactions typically fall into two categories: direct and indirect. In the direct category, two substances interact with each other, often causing a potent reaction. In contrast, the indirect category involves one substance altering how the body processes another, affecting factors like absorption, metabolism, or transportation throughout the body.

Consider blood thinners and aspirin, for instance. Individually, they're safe, each working to prevent blood clots in their own way. Blood thinners hinder the formation of clotting factors, while aspirin stops blood cells from clumping together to form clots. But when taken together, they create a dangerous synergy, potentially preventing blood clotting to a dangerous extent, which could lead to internal bleeding.

This isn't just limited to medications that are independently safe. Sometimes, interactions occur between drugs that are harmful on their own, like cocaine and heroin. Although they might seem to counteract each other's effects, they actually create a deadly combo. Cocaine, a stimulant, raises oxygen demand in the body due to increased heart rate, while heroin, a depressant, reduces oxygen supply by slowing breathing. This toxic duo can strain organs, leading to respiratory failure and, in some cases, death.

Now, let's delve into a peculiar pairing – grapefruit

juice and certain cholesterol-lowering drugs called statins. This interaction revolves around the intricate world of drug metabolism. You see, your liver has a crew of enzymes tasked with breaking down substances that enter your body. These enzymes can either activate drugs or deactivate harmful compounds.

Here's where grapefruit juice comes into play. It shares an enzyme with statins, and when you consume grapefruit juice while taking these medications, it's like a party crasher stealing the spotlight. Grapefruit grabs the enzyme's attention, leaving less of it available to break down statins. As a result, the concentration of the drug in your bloodstream can skyrocket, potentially causing kidney failure.

But grapefruit juice isn't the only culprit. Alcohol can also throw a wrench into the mix by altering the enzyme responsible for breaking down acetaminophen, the active ingredient in pain relievers like Tylenol. Typically, at the recommended dose, there's not enough of a toxic byproduct to cause harm. However, heavy drinking can increase the production of this toxic substance, putting your liver at risk, even with a usually safe dose of acetaminophen.

And let's not forget about herbal remedies like St. John's wort. It can speed up the production of a specific enzyme in your liver. While this might sound harmless, it can lead to the rapid metabolism of certain drugs, preventing them from having their intended therapeutic effects.

With countless potential interactions, navigating this minefield may seem impossible. But fear not, because science is racing to our rescue. Some brilliant minds are developing AI programs that can predict the side effects of drug interactions before they occur. These programs use information about the intricate web of protein interactions within your body, offering us a glimpse into the future of drug safety.

Additionally, supercomputers are being employed to identify potential interactions for new drugs while they're still in development. With these advancements, we're moving closer to a world where the shadowy dangers of drug interactions become a thing of the past.

So, next time you reach for that medication or consider pairing it with something else, remember the unseen threats that can lurk in the background. Knowledge is your greatest weapon in this battle, and with the help of science, we can make informed choices that keep us safe from these hidden dangers. Stay curious, stay vigilant, and, above all, stay safe.

## Act fast, save lives. Cerebral strokes.

Picture this: every two seconds, somewhere around the globe, someone's life takes an unexpected turn. It's like a sudden detour on the road of life. What happens? They experience a stroke, and it's a lot more common than you might think. In fact, one out of every six people will face this challenge at some point in their lives.

Now, let's dive into what exactly happens when a stroke strikes. Our brains are incredible, consuming over 20% of the oxygen in our blood, even though they make up just 2% of our body mass. That's a lot of oxygen! To fuel our brains, we have a network of blood vessels, kind of like highways, delivering that vital oxygen.

But here's the catch: sometimes, these "highways" get blocked. Imagine a traffic jam during rush hour. In the world of strokes, there are two main types. First, we have hemorrhagic strokes, which are like a burst water pipe, causing blood to leak out. The second and more common type is ischemic strokes. These are like a roadblock in our brain's blood vessels.

But why do these roadblocks happen? Well, sometimes, it's because of a tricky situation in our hearts. Imagine your heart is a DJ, setting the rhythm for a party. If it starts playing a weird beat, it can make platelets and clotting factors come together, just like people coming together on the dance floor.

This can create a clot, which is like a sticky ball, and it can travel through your bloodstream like a traveler looking for adventure. Eventually, it might get stuck in one of the brain's blood vessels, and that's when trouble strikes.

Now, our brains are silent workers. They don't feel pain like our fingers or toes. But when they're not getting enough oxygen, they start sending out distress signals. It's like your brain sending out an SOS message. If the area responsible for speech is affected, you might notice slurred words. If it controls your muscles, one side of your body might weaken.

Here's where things get crucial: time is of the essence. The quicker you get medical help, the better. The first line of treatment is an intravenous medication called Tissue Plasminogen Activator, which can break up the blood clot and allow blood to flow again in the compromised artery. If it's delivered within a few hours, this medication greatly increases the chance of surviving the stroke and avoiding permanent consequences. If tissue plasminogen activator cannot be given because the patient is on certain medications, has history of major bleeding, or the clot is particularly large, doctors can perform a procedure called an endovascular thrombectomy. Imagine a tiny superhero robot navigating through your blood vessels to remove the clot like a master locksmith picking a lock.

Now, how can you be a hero in this story? Remember the FAST test: F for facial drooping, A
for arm weakness, S for speech difficulties, and T for time. If you spot any of these signs in someone, don't wait! Call for help immediately, because acting fast can save lives.

So, strokes may be like unexpected detours, but with quick action and the right treatment, the road to recovery can be a lot smoother. Stay vigilant, stay informed, and remember that every second counts when it comes to strokes!

## Thyroid: The Metabolism Maestro in Your Body

Deep in your neck, there's a small but mighty organ called the thyroid, and it's a bit like the boss of your body. Its main job is to make sure all your cells are doing their work properly. It's like a manager, and it uses special messengers called hormones to tell your cells what to do.

Inside the thyroid, there are these little parts called lobules, and each of them has tiny cells called follicles. These follicles store the hormones that the thyroid sends out into your blood. Two of the most important hormones it makes are called thyroxine and triiodothyronine, but you can just call them T3 and T4 for short.

These hormones are like emails or text messages that your thyroid sends to all the cells in your body. They tell the cells when to use oxygen and nutrients, which keeps your metabolism going. Metabolism is like all the little reactions inside your cells that give you energy.

So when you need more energy, your thyroid sends out more hormones, and that makes your heart beat faster, your cells work harder, and your body breaks down food faster. It's like getting a little energy boost!

But here's the cool part: your thyroid doesn't do all of this on its own. It gets orders from another part of your brain called the pituitary gland. The pituitary gland checks if the hormone levels in your blood are just right. If they're too low or too high, it sends a message to the thyroid to fix it.

But sometimes, things can go a bit haywire. If your thyroid starts sending out too many hormones, it's like it's giving your cells too many instructions at once. This can make your cells work too fast, and that's called hyperthyroidism. When that happens, you might feel hungry, lose weight quickly, feel too hot, and have trouble sleeping.

On the other hand, if your thyroid doesn't send out enough hormones, it's like your cells aren't getting enough messages. That's called hypothyroidism, and it can make you gain weight, feel sluggish, cold, and a bit sad.

But the good news is, there are treatments to help your thyroid get back on track and keep your body working just right. Even though it's a small organ, the thyroid does a big job, and it helps keep everything in your body running smoothly, even if you don't always notice it!

## What would happen if you didn´t sleep?

Back in 1965, a 17-year-old high school student named Randy Garner did something really unusual. He stayed awake for a really long time, 11 days to be exact, just to see how his body would react without sleep. It's like when you try an experiment to see what happens, but this one was all about sleep.

On the second day of his experiment, Randy's eyes stopped working properly. They couldn't focus on things. Then, he lost the ability to feel and recognize objects by touching them. Things got even worse on the third day when he became grumpy and couldn't move properly. By the end of his no-sleep adventure, he had a hard time concentrating, remembering things, and even started seeing things that weren't really there.

Luckily, Randy didn't have any long-term problems from this, but for some people, not getting enough sleep can be really bad. We're still figuring out why we need sleep, but we do know it's super important. Adults need about 7 to 8 hours of sleep each night, and teenagers need even more, about 10 hours.

When it's time to sleep, our bodies send signals to our brain, saying, "Hey, we're tired!" Plus, the environment around us gets darker at night, which also tells our brain it's time to sleep. Then, special chemicals in our body, like adenosine and melatonin, make us start feeling sleepy.

When we sleep, our body goes through different stages, like a movie with different scenes. During one of these stages, called non-REM sleep, our body gets busy repairing our DNA and fixing up our muscles and organs for the next day.

But here's the tricky part: lots of people don't get enough sleep. In the United States, around 30% of grown-ups and a whopping 66% of teenagers aren't getting the sleep they need. And this isn't just a small problem. Not getting enough sleep can mess with our learning, memory, mood, and how fast we react to things.

It can even make our bodies feel bad, like causing inflammation, high blood pressure, and even making us see things that aren't real. In some really sad cases, people have even died because they stayed awake for too long. Like a soccer fan who stayed up for 48 hours to watch a game and had a stroke.

There's a rare condition called fatal familial insomnia where people can't sleep at all, and it gets worse over time, leading to dementia and, eventually, death. So, you can see that sleep is super important for our bodies and our brains to work properly.

Scientists think that when we're awake, our brain cells create waste products, kind of like trash that piles up during the day. One of these waste products is called adenosine, and it makes us feel more and more tired as it builds up. That's why caffeine, like in coffee, works by blocking the sleepy effects of adenosine.

Other waste products also collect in our brains during the day. If they aren't cleaned up, they can overload our brain and make us feel bad when we don't get enough sleep. But here's the cool part: when we do sleep, our brain has a special system to clean up all that mess.

It's called the glymphatic system, and it uses a special fluid to wash away the waste products. Imagine it like a cleaning crew that comes in at night to tidy up your brain. Scientists also recently found special vessels in the brain that help with this cleanup job.

So, even though we're still learning about all the amazing things that happen when we sleep, one thing is clear: getting a good night's sleep is super important if we want to stay healthy and feel our best!

## The cancer gene that is inside everyone

Alright, imagine your body is like a car on the road, and your cells are the drivers. Normally, your body is pretty good at making sure the cells in your body don't go too fast. But sometimes, something goes wrong, like when the brakes in a car stop working. In the world of your body, we call this "cancer."

So, what happens when the "brakes" in your body, which are supposed to control how fast your cells divide, stop working? Well, your cells start dividing super-fast, like they're in a big hurry. This can lead to something called "mutations," which are like mistakes in the instructions that tell your cells what to do.

Imagine your cells as workers in a factory, and these mutations make them forget their job. They start doing things they're not supposed to, and that can create something called a "tumor," which is like a big traffic jam in your body. These tumors can mess up how your body works, like how you breathe or digest your food, and that can be really bad.

Now, your body has some special genes that act like traffic cops. One of these genes is called "BRCA1," which stands for "breast cancer susceptibility gene 1." It's like the super boss of the factory, making sure everything goes smoothly. BRCA1 helps fix those mistakes in your cell's instructions (DNA) when they happen.

Here's the thing: you have two copies of this BRCA1 gene in every cell, one from your mom and one from your dad. It's like having a backup plan. But not all BRCA1 genes are the same. Some are better at fixing mistakes than others. So, some people are born with better "traffic cops" than others.

But if a BRCA1 gene doesn't work because of a mutation, it's like the traffic cops taking a break. Cells with damaged instructions can start dividing, and as they do, they might make even more mistakes. This can lead to the cells becoming all mixed up and not doing their normal job in your body's "factory." And that's when there's a higher chance they could turn into cancer cells.

So, while we all have genes like BRCA1 that can cause cancer, it's only when these genes don't do their job properly that we run into trouble. Having a BRCA1 gene that doesn't work right can make you more likely to get cancer, kind of like how driving a car with bad brakes makes accidents more likely.

**Have you ever wondered how we smell?**

Let's dive into the fascinating world of your sense of smell. It's actually the first sense you use when you're born, and it's pretty important. Think about the last time you took a deep breath through your nose – that's your sense of smell at work!

Your nose is like a super detective, and it can detect around 10,000 different smells when you're all grown up. Here's how it all happens: tiny smell molecules go up your nose when you sniff the air. Most of your nose is like a filter, making sure the air you breathe is clean before it reaches your lungs. But at the very back of your nose, there's a special area called the olfactory epithelium. It's like a little patch of skin that's super important for your sense of smell.

Inside this olfactory epithelium are olfactory receptor cells, which are like the taste buds of your nose. When those smell molecules reach the back of your nose, they get stuck in a layer of gooey stuff called mucus that covers the olfactory epithelium. As they dissolve in the mucus, they stick to the olfactory receptor cells, which then send signals to your brain.

By the way, you can tell how good an animal's sense of smell is by checking the size of its olfactory epithelium. For example, a dog's olfactory epithelium is 20 times bigger than ours – they're like smell experts!

But here's something scientists still puzzle over: our olfactory epithelium is pigmented, which means it has color, but we're not exactly sure why. And now, let's get into how you tell the difference between smells. Your brain has a whopping 40 million different olfactory receptor neurons. So when you smell something, like a delicious pie or a fragrant flower, your brain gets a combination of signals from these neurons. It's like a secret code for each smell!

These different combinations of signals help you detect a huge variety of smells. Plus, your olfactory neurons are always fresh and ready for action. They're the only neurons in your body that get replaced regularly, every four to eight weeks.

When these neurons are triggered, the signals travel through a bundle called the olfactory tract to different parts of your brain. This differs from how your eyes and ears work – their signals go to a middleman in the brain and then get sent to other parts. But smell, because it's one of the oldest senses in our history, goes directly to different brain regions. This is why smells can make you feel scared, bring back memories, or even make your mouth water for some tasty food.

Here's a cool fact: not everyone smells the same things in the same way! Take asparagus, for example. After some people eat it, their pee has a distinct smell, but not everyone notices it. There are other scents that smell differently to different people, too, like a chemical called androsinone, which can smell like vanilla to some and like sweaty urine to others. That's why some pigs get castrated to avoid making androsinone in their

meat – so it doesn't taste funny to everyone.

But there's more to the story. Some people can't smell anything at all, and this is called anosmia. There are about a hundred known examples of this. It can happen because someone is born without a sense of smell, or they might lose it after an accident or during an illness. Sometimes, when your olfactory epithelium gets swollen or infected, like when you have a bad cold, it can mess with your sense of smell too.

But here's the twist: not being able to smell can affect your sense of taste as well. See, when you chew your food, air carries the smell of your food up your nose. Those scents hit your olfactory epithelium and tell your brain a lot about what you're eating. So, if you can't smell, you lose the ability to taste all those fancy flavors. Instead, you're left with just the basic tastes your taste buds can detect – sweet, salty, bitter, sour, and savory.

So next time you catch a whiff of something delicious, like a yummy dessert or a tasty meal, remember it's your super-smart nose and brain working together to help you enjoy it. And be thankful that you can, because smelling and tasting are pretty awesome!

## Why is it so hard to cure HIV?

Allow me to embark on a fascinating journey back to the year 2008, a year that witnessed something truly extraordinary unfold. A man achieved the seemingly impossible: he was cured of HIV, a feat previously unheard of in the annals of over 70 million HIV cases. Yet, the enigma surrounding this cure persists, shrouded in a veil of uncertainty. We are left pondering why we can triumph over diseases like malaria and hepatitis C, but HIV remains an elusive adversary, slipping through our grasp?

Let us embark on a quest for understanding, starting with the insidious manner in which HIV infiltrates the human body, stealthily progressing into the dreaded condition known as AIDS. The transmission of this virus hinges on exchanges of bodily fluids, with unprotected sexual encounters and the sharing of contaminated needles ranking as the primary modes of transmission.

The silver lining in this narrative, however, lies in the fact that HIV does not possess the sinister capability to spread through the air we breathe, the water we drink, or even casual contact with others. It's an equal opportunity intruder, indiscriminately affecting individuals across age, sexual orientation, gender, and race. Once it infiltrates the human fortress, HIV targets a specific type of immune cell known as helper T cells, which play a vital role in safeguarding our bodies against bacterial and fungal adversaries.

As we delve deeper into the mysteries of HIV, we begin to unravel the complexities that have confounded scientists and medical practitioners alike, offering a glimpse into the ongoing quest to conquer this formidable foe. HIV is a retrovirus, which means it can write its genetic code into the genome of infected cells, co-opting them into making more copies of itself. During the first stage of HIV infection, the virus replicates within helper T cells, destroying many of them in the process.

During this stage, patients often experience flu-like symptoms but are typically not yet in mortal danger. However, for a period ranging from a few months to several years, during which time the patient may look and feel completely healthy, the virus continues to replicate and destroy T cells.

When T-cell counts drop too low, patients are in serious danger of contracting deadly infections that healthy immune systems can normally handle. This stage of HIV infection is known as AIDS. The good news is, there are drugs that are highly effective at managing levels of HIV and preventing T cell counts from getting low enough for the disease to progress to AIDS.

The second, equally poignant challenge casts a shadow on our global canvas. Regrettably, not every corner of our world enjoys equal access to the therapies that could offer salvation. Inequality in healthcare access remains a harsh reality, leaving countless individuals without the means to embrace the life-extending potential of these treatments. It's a stark reminder that while we make strides in our battle against HIV, the battle for equitable access to healthcare rages on, a battle that remains far from won.

In sub-Saharan Africa, which accounts for over 70% of HIV patients worldwide, antiretrovirals reached only about 1 in 3 HIV -positive patients in 2012. There is no easy answer to this problem. A mix of political, economic, and cultural barriers makes effective prevention and treatment difficult.

And even in the US, HIV still claims more than 10,000 lives per year. However, there is ample cause for hope. Researchers may be closer than ever to developing a true cure. One research approach involves using a drug to activate all cells harboring the HIV genetic information.

This would both destroy those cells and flush the virus out into the open, where our current drugs are effective. Another is looking to use genetic tools to cut the HIV DNA out of cells' genomes altogether.

And while one cure out of 70 million cases may seem like terrible odds, one is immeasurably better than zero. We now know that a cure is possible, and that may give us what we need to beat HIV for good.

# The Complex World of Eating Disorders

In the intricate tapestry of human health, eating disorders stand out as some of the most enigmatic and challenging conditions to understand and treat. Despite affecting around 10% of the global population at some point in their lives, these disorders are often shrouded in misconceptions and a lack of comprehensive understanding. This gap in knowledge not only hampers effective treatment but also leaves those affected and their loved ones grappling in the dark for solutions and support.

Eating disorders, encompassing a spectrum of psychiatric conditions, manifest in behaviors like restricting food intake, binging, and purging. These patterns can appear in various combinations, making each case unique. Anorexia nervosa, for instance, is characterized by severe food restriction, while bulimia nervosa involves cycles of binge eating followed by purging. Crucially, these disorders are not discernible through weight alone; they can afflict individuals across the weight spectrum, often inflicting invisible yet severe long-term health consequences.

At their core, eating disorders are psychiatric illnesses, deeply rooted in disruptions to self-perception and critical self-assessment. Many who suffer from these conditions report a heightened sense of self-critique and often use eating patterns as a means to exert control over an internal sense of turmoil. The causes of eating disorders are complex and multifaceted, involving a blend of genetic predispositions and environmental factors. Mental health issues like depression and anxiety often intertwine with these disorders, while societal pressures, including weight stigma and body image dissatisfaction, play significant roles.

Contrary to popular belief, eating disorders are not exclusive to women; they affect people of all genders. Adolescence, a critical period for identity and self-esteem development, is a particularly vulnerable time for the onset of these disorders. Despite their complexity, eating disorders are treatable, and many individuals recover fully with appropriate intervention. However, early detection and treatment are crucial, and sadly, less than half of those affected seek and receive the help they need.

Treatment for eating disorders typically involves a holistic approach, combining nutritional counseling, various psychotherapies, and sometimes medication. Cognitive-behavioral therapy and family-based therapy are among the evidence-based treatments that have shown effectiveness. These therapies aim to equip individuals with the skills to address the psychological underpinnings of their eating behaviors. For those who do not respond to traditional treatments, researchers are exploring alternative methods, such as transcranial magnetic stimulation.

The journey through an eating disorder can be a harrowing one, marked by a profound sense of powerlessness. Yet, through education and awareness, individuals, families, and communities can begin to dismantle the stigma surrounding these conditions, improving access to treatment and support. In understanding the complexities of eating disorders, we take a vital step toward shining a light on these shadowed paths, offering hope and guidance to those navigating this challenging terrain.

## Nourishing the Brain's Inner Universe

Embark on a journey into the depths of your brain, a voyage to unravel the intricate relationship between the food you eat and the vast expanse of your cerebral landscape. Picture your brain, not as a mere organ, but as a complex ecosystem, thriving on the nutrients you consume. If you could strip away all its moisture and break it down to its core components, you'd find that a significant portion of your dehydrated brain is composed of fats, or lipids, as scientists refer to them.

Venturing further into this cerebral terrain, you'd encounter a rich tapestry of proteins and amino acids, traces of vital micronutrients, and the ever-essential glucose, the fuel that powers the cognitive machinery. However, the brain is more than just a collection of nutrients. It's a dynamic entity where each component plays a distinct role, shaping your thoughts, emotions, and the energy that courses through your mind.

The foods you consume cast a direct influence on your brain's performance and well-being. Among the fats in your brain, Omega 3 and 6 fatty acids stand out as crucial players. These essential fats, linked to staving off degenerative brain conditions, must be sourced from your diet.

Consuming omega-rich foods like nuts, seeds, and fatty fish is vital for the formation and upkeep of cell membranes. Yet, it's not just about the good fats. The long-term intake of other fats, such as trans and saturated fats, can potentially impair

brain health.

Proteins and amino acids, the foundational nutrients of growth and development, also play a pivotal role in modulating our emotions and actions. They are the precursors to neurotransmitters, the brain's chemical messengers. These neurotransmitters influence a myriad of functions, from mood and sleep to alertness and appetite. This is why certain foods can induce a sense of calm or heightened alertness.

The complex interplay of compounds in our diet can stimulate brain cells to release mood-altering chemicals like norepinephrine, dopamine, and serotonin. It's a delicate dance of elements, where each nutrient contributes to the grand performance of the brain.

In this exploration of the brain's nutritional universe, we begin to understand how our dietary choices resonate through the corridors of our minds.

Each meal, each bite, is not just sustenance but a source of influence, shaping the very essence of our thoughts and feelings. "Mindful Meals: Nourishing the Brain's Inner Universe" is more than a story of food and the brain; it's a narrative about the profound connections between what we eat and who we are, at our very core.

## Echoes of Silence: Navigating the Sonic World Without Losing Sound

In the aftermath of an exhilarating Taylor Swift concert, Jade found herself enveloped in a world of muffled sounds and persistent ringing. This unexpected turn of events led her down a path of discovery, seeking answers to the sudden shift in her auditory experience. The concert, a symphony of sound and emotion, had unknowingly ushered her into the complex realm of auditory health.

Sound, in its essence, is a vibration that travels through air, much like ripples in a pond. Our ears, those intricate organs, are finely tuned to interpret these vibrations, translating them into the rich tapestry of sounds we experience daily. The journey of sound begins as it enters the ear canal, striking the eardrum, and setting in motion the ossicular chain, a trio of tiny bones that amplify these vibrations into the cochlea.

Within the cochlea, a fluid wave is generated, moving the basilar membrane and its delicate hair cells. These hair cells, with their fine stereocilia, are the critical translators, converting mechanical vibrations into electrical signals for the brain to interpret as sound. However, these microscopic hair cells are also remarkably fragile, susceptible to damage from excessive volume and prolonged exposure to sound.

The concert's sonic tidal wave, measured in decibels, had exerted immense pressure on Jade's hair cells. Prolonged exposure to sounds above 120 decibels can irreparably damage these cells, leading to permanent hearing loss. Even at lower volumes, extended exposure can cause temporary threshold shifts, where hearing becomes muffled as hair cells and their supporting tissue swell.

Jade's experience was a classic case of temporary threshold shift, a common condition that often resolves with time and avoidance of further auditory stress. However, repeated exposure to high sound levels can lead to chronic conditions like tinnitus or difficulty discerning speech in noisy environments. These overworked hair cells can produce reactive oxygen species, harmful molecules that cause lasting damage to the inner ear.

To safeguard against hearing loss, it's crucial to manage exposure to loud sounds. Using earbuds or headphones at 80% volume or lower, especially for prolonged periods, can significantly reduce the risk. Noise-isolating headphones are another effective tool, allowing for lower volume listening. Regular hearing checkups, much like dental or vision exams, are essential in maintaining auditory health.

In regions where access to audiologists is limited, innovative solutions are emerging. Portable hearing tests and user-friendly apps are being developed to bring essential hearing care to remote communities. These initiatives are transforming the landscape of auditory health, ensuring that the joy of sound remains accessible
to all.
At the heart of this story is a simple yet powerful message: our hearing is a precious gift, one that requires mindful protection. Whether at a concert or in everyday life, the right precautions, like properly fitted earplugs, can make all the difference. By understanding and respecting the limits of our auditory system, we can continue to enjoy the vibrant world of sound without sacrificing the health of our ears..

## Chemotherapy: The Superhero Team in the Fight Against Cancer

In the United States, cancer stands as the second leading cause of death, accounting for nearly 21.7% of all deaths annually. When faced with this formidable adversary, the most effective treatment becomes a paramount concern. While surgery and radiation are potent tools, effective in specific scenarios like early-stage tumors, they fall short when cancer metastasizes. This is where chemotherapy, akin to a superhero team, enters the fray.

Chemotherapy involves a diverse array of drugs, each akin to a superhero with unique abilities, administered through an injection into the bloodstream. These drugs embark on a mission throughout the body, seeking out elusive cancer cells hidden in various tissues and organs.

The primary strategy of these superhero drugs is to target the cancer cells' DNA, their instruction manual. By disrupting the DNA, akin to messing up a recipe, the cells lose their ability to function and grow, leading to their eventual demise. Some chemotherapy agents achieve this by gluing parts of the DNA together, preventing it from replicating, while others inhibit a key cellular worker, topoisomerase, essential for DNA maintenance. As a result, the cancer cells, unable to sustain themselves, opt for cellular suicide.

Another group within this superhero team are the mitotic inhibitors. These agents target a specific phase in the cell cycle called mitosis, the process of cell division. By halting the cell cycle during mitosis, much like stopping a Ferris wheel mid-rotation, these drugs prevent cancer cells from proliferating. Since cancer cells typically grow faster than normal cells, they are more likely to be caught in the mitosis phase and thus are more susceptible to these inhibitors.

However, this approach is not without its challenges. Mitotic inhibitors can also affect fast-growing normal cells, such as those in the intestines, skin, and hair, leading to side effects like hair loss, skin rashes, and gastrointestinal discomfort. Moreover, not all cancers grow rapidly, making some less responsive to mitotic inhibitors. This variability necessitates a combination of treatments, employing different mechanisms to combat various types of cancer effectively.

In summary, chemotherapy is like deploying a team of superheroes with diverse powers to disrupt the inner workings of cancer cells. While the battle is tough and often accompanied by collateral damage, this approach remains a cornerstone in the fight against cancer, offering hope and a fighting chance to those afflicted..

## The Allure of Asymmetry: Unraveling the Mysteries of the Human Body

In the natural world, symmetry is often celebrated for its balance and harmony, evident in the perfect shapes of leaves and the mirrored patterns of butterfly wings. However, it's the peculiar charm of asymmetry that captivates us in many forms of life, from the uneven claws of lobsters to the spiraling of seashells. This asymmetry is not just an external phenomenon; it's intricately woven into the very fabric of our being, especially evident in the human body.

While the human body appears symmetrical on the outside, a deeper look reveals a different story. Our vital organs are arranged asymmetrically: the heart, stomach, spleen, and pancreas lean towards the left, while the gallbladder and most of the liver sit on the right. Even our lungs and brain exhibit asymmetry, with differing lobes and functions. This internal asymmetry is crucial for our survival, as conditions like situs inversus, where organ positions are mirrored, can lead to severe health complications.

The origin of this asymmetry is a fascinating tale that begins at the embryonic stage. Initially, an embryo appears identical on both sides. The key to asymmetry lies in a small structure called the node, lined with tiny, synchronously rotating hairs called cilia.

These cilia create a fluid flow from right to left across the node, triggering specific genes on the embryo's left side. These genes instruct cells to produce certain proteins, leading to chemical differences between the right and left sides, even though they appear identical.

The heart is the first organ to exhibit asymmetry, starting as a straight tube that bends and rotates towards the right, eventually forming the asymmetric heart we know. Other major organs follow, emerging from a central tube and growing towards their designated positions. Interestingly, some organisms, like pigs, lack these embryonic cilia yet still develop asymmetric organs, suggesting a deeper, intrinsic cellular asymmetry.

Zooming in further, we find that many of the basic building blocks of cells, such as nucleic acids, proteins, and sugars, are inherently asymmetric. Proteins, with their complex shapes, dictate cell migration and the direction of embryonic cilia twirl. This asymmetry at the molecular level, known as chirality, is akin to the difference between our right and left hands – similar in appearance but not identical.

In conclusion, while symmetry may capture our eyes with its beauty, asymmetry holds a deeper allure. It's found in the graceful swirls of nature, the organized complexity of our bodies, and the striking imperfections that make life diverse and fascinating.

Asymmetry in the human body is not just a quirk but a fundamental aspect of our existence, reflecting the intricate and beautiful tapestry of life.

## Demystifying the Immune System: Beyond the Hype of 'Boosting

The quest to boost the immune system is a common pursuit, especially in a world where products like turmeric, ginger shots, elderberry syrup, and vitamin C tablets are touted as immune-boosting miracles. However, the truth about the immune system is more complex than simply strengthening it like a muscle through antioxidants and supplements.

The immune system is a sophisticated network of cells, tissues, and organs, functioning through two primary mechanisms: innate immunity and adaptive immunity. Innate immunity acts as the body's first line of defense, akin to a bouncer at a club's door, preventing or neutralizing pathogens before they cause harm. This includes physical barriers like skin and mucous membranes, as well as general immune responses.

If a pathogen breaches these defenses, the adaptive immune system comes into play. This system is more specialized and targeted, responding to specific antigens, which are unique proteins on the surface of pathogens. The adaptive immune system employs lymphocytes, specialized white blood cells, to attack these invaders. Remarkably, it also has a memory, allowing it to recognize and respond more effectively to pathogens it has encountered before.

The concept of 'boosting' the immune system is

problematic because it oversimplifies this intricate system. For instance, boosting one aspect, like histamine, could lead to excessive itching, while overstimulating T and B cells might trigger autoimmune responses. The immune system is more akin to a garden with diverse components, each requiring a delicate balance of care.

A healthy, balanced diet typically provides all the necessary nutrients for the immune system to function optimally. Excess intake of certain vitamins doesn't enhance immune function; the body simply excretes what it doesn't need. Vitamin supplements are beneficial only in cases of genuine deficiency. In fact, unnecessary supplementation can sometimes have adverse effects.

While the immune system can malfunction, leading to allergies, autoimmune disorders, or failure to eliminate abnormal cells, these issues are complex and not fully understood. They certainly aren't solvable by any 'miracle' immune-boosting pill.

However, one intervention has consistently proven beneficial for the immune system: vaccines. Vaccines are ingenious in their simplicity and effectiveness. They introduce a weakened or inactive part of a pathogen, including its antigen, to the body. This triggers the production of antibodies without the need to experience the actual illness.

Vaccines don't boost the immune system indiscriminately; instead, they prepare it to
respond swiftly and robustly to specific pathogens.
Maintaining a healthy immune system isn't about seeking a magic solution. It involves getting recommended vaccinations, eating a balanced diet, avoiding smoking, and ensuring adequate sleep. Letting the immune system function as it's designed to, without unnecessary interference, is often the best approach to staying healthy.

**The Myth of Detox: Understanding the True Protectors of Our Body**

The allure of detox diets and cleanses, ranging from charcoal-infused lemonades to detox teas, is undeniable in our quest for health. However, the effectiveness of these products in actually 'detoxifying' the body is a misconception rooted in a misunderstanding of our body's natural processes.

The concept of purification is not new; it has been intertwined with medicine and religion for thousands of years. Ancient practices like bloodletting, purging, and fasting were believed to cleanse the body of toxins and restore humoral balance. Fast forward to modern times, and the wellness industry has repackaged this age-old idea of detoxification, originally used in medical contexts for drug and alcohol dependency, into a lucrative market of cleansing regimens.

The notion of detox diets is often compared to flushing out a clogged pipe, but this analogy fails to recognize the complexity and efficiency of the liver, our body's natural detoxifier. The liver, a three-pound organ in the upper right abdomen, is a multitasking powerhouse. It plays a crucial role in immune support, blood clotting, cholesterol and hormone production, and, most importantly, processing harmful substances.

The liver functions like a sophisticated factory, transforming nutrients from our intake into usable forms or expelling them as waste. When it encounters alcohol, for instance, the liver breaks it down in a multi-step process, converting it into less harmful substances that the body can easily handle.

Popular cleanses, like cayenne pepper or lemon juice drinks, are processed by the liver in the same way as other foods and drinks. The liver extracts useful nutrients and discards the rest as waste. While some may experience temporary weight loss from these cleanses due to reduced food intake, the risks include potential starvation mode, electrolyte imbalance, and disruption of intestinal flora and bowel function.

Maintaining liver health is crucial, and the best ways to do so are through lifestyle choices: avoiding smoking, eating a balanced diet, regular exercise, and sufficient sleep. Liver-specific precautions include moderate alcohol consumption, careful use of medications, vaccination against hepatitis B, and screening for hepatitis C. Additionally, caution is advised with supplements, especially those marketed for bodybuilding or weight loss, as they can cause liver damage.

The concept of detox diets as a form of self-care is misleading. True self-care involves understanding our bodies and making informed decisions based on this knowledge. Our liver, along with other organs, efficiently performs detoxification daily, rendering these marketed detox products unnecessary. The best approach to health is to support our body's natural processes through healthy lifestyle choices.

## Scars: The Story of Healing and Resilience Written on Our Skin

Scars are more than just marks on our skin; they are the tangible remnants of our body's remarkable healing process. Whether from a childhood fall, a surgical procedure, or a deliberate act in certain cultures, scars narrate stories of resilience and recovery.

When we examine healthy skin tissue under a microscope, we find cells performing various functions, interconnected by an extracellular matrix (ECM). This ECM, primarily composed of structural proteins like collagen, is secreted by fibroblast cells. It facilitates nutrient transportation, cell communication, and adhesion. However, when a deep wound disrupts this intricate arrangement, the healing process alters the skin's original structure.

During wound healing, collagen is redeposited at the site. Unlike the basket-weave pattern of healthy tissue, this new ECM aligns in a single direction. This alignment hampers intercellular processes and diminishes the skin's durability and elasticity. The healed area has a higher proportion of ECM, compromising its functionality.

Scar tissue impacts the skin's primary roles, such as sweat production, temperature regulation, and hair growth. It is more fragile and sensitive to temperature and sensation changes. Keeping the scarred area moist can aid in healing. This phenomenon, known as fibrosis, is not exclusive to the skin. It can occur in various organs, leading to conditions like cystic fibrosis in the pancreas and pulmonary fibrosis in the lungs. In the heart, scarring post-heart attack can hinder its function, potentially causing further complications.

Despite retaining some original functions, scar tissue is inherently inferior to the native tissue it replaces. However, there is hope in the horizon. Medical research is delving into the mechanisms behind fibroblast cells' excessive collagen secretion and exploring ways to encourage other cells to regenerate and repopulate damaged tissue. This understanding could revolutionize wound healing and scar formation, potentially transforming the way we address the aftermath of injuries.

Until such advancements are realized, our scars serve as reminders of our body's ability to heal and the experiences that shaped us. They are not just blemishes but symbols of our journey through life, each one holding a unique story of survival and resilience.

## The Dynamics of Blood Pressure: A Journey Through Our Circulatory System

Blood pressure is a vital force in our circulatory system, a phenomenon as dynamic as it is crucial. Imagine the vast network of blood vessels in your body, stretching an astonishing 95,000 kilometers, circulating about 7,500 liters of blood daily. This blood, the same four or five liters recycled repeatedly, is the lifeline delivering oxygen and nutrients to every tissue.

Blood pressure is the force exerted by this blood against the muscular walls of our blood vessels. It fluctuates with the heartbeat, reaching its peak during systole when the heart contracts to pump blood through the arteries. This peak is known as systolic blood pressure. Between beats, as the heart rests, blood pressure drops to its lowest point, called diastolic pressure. A healthy individual typically has a systolic pressure between 90 and 120 millimeters of mercury and a diastolic pressure between 60 and 80, making a normal reading slightly less than 120 over 80.

Several factors can influence blood pressure. For instance, thicker blood requires more force to move, prompting the heart to pump harder. A high-salt diet can lead to water retention, increasing blood volume and, consequently, blood pressure. Stress triggers the release of hormones like epinephrine and norepinephrine, constricting key blood vessels and raising pressure.

Blood vessels, resilient due to elastic fibers in their walls, usually handle these fluctuations well. However, consistently high blood pressure, known as hypertension (typically above 140 over 90), poses significant risks. It can cause small tears in arterial walls, leading to inflammation and the accumulation of white blood cells, fat, and cholesterol. This buildup, known as atherosclerosis, can stiffen and thicken the arterial walls.

The consequences of atherosclerosis can be severe. A ruptured plaque can lead to blood clots, obstructing blood flow. In the heart, this blockage can cause a heart attack, and in the brain, it can result in a stroke. Treatments like angioplasty, where a balloon catheter is used to open narrowed vessels, or the placement of a stent, can alleviate these blockages.

Our arteries, tasked with staying flexible under constant pressure, face challenges from the sticky substances in the blood and the relentless beating of the heart, about 70 times a minute and over two and a half billion times in an average lifetime. Despite these immense pressures, our circulatory system is remarkably equipped to handle the task, ensuring that life-sustaining blood flows unimpeded throughout our body.

## Steroids: The Double-Edged Sword of Performance Enhancement

Steroids, often associated with sports and bodybuilding, are substances similar to testosterone, the hormone largely responsible for muscle growth. Over 3 million Americans have used steroids, driven by the desire to enhance physical appearance and athletic performance. But what exactly happens in your body when you take steroids, and what are the risks involved?

In the context of muscle building, steroids are used to amplify the natural process of muscle repair and growth. Normally, when muscles are stressed during exercise, they undergo repair through the formation of new protein strands, leading to increased muscle size. Testosterone plays a key role in this process by enhancing protein synthesis. Men, typically having higher testosterone levels, generally possess larger muscle mass compared to women.

Steroids mimic natural testosterone, aiming to boost muscle growth and performance. They work by entering cells and binding to androgen receptors, which then activate genes responsible for protein synthesis. This process significantly increases muscle cell nuclei, enhancing muscle growth while also inhibiting cortisol, a molecule that promotes the breakdown of proteins.

However, the use of steroids for recreational purposes differs significantly from medical applications. Recreational users often consume much higher doses than medically prescribed, leading to a range of side effects and health risks. While steroids can aid muscle growth and recovery, and are beneficial in medical contexts like aiding patients with AIDS, cancer, or severe burns, their recreational use carries significant risks.

Steroids can alter behavior, potentially leading to 'roid rage' – episodes of anger and aggression. They are particularly risky for adolescents, as they can disrupt normal growth patterns. Studies have shown increased manic and depressive behaviors in steroid users, and animal studies indicate heightened aggression.

The impact on sexual health is also notable. In women, steroids can disrupt the estrogen cycle, leading to decreased sexual drive and masculinization effects like deeper voices and increased body hair. In men, steroids can cause sperm abnormalities, decreased sperm count, and reduced natural hormone production, leading to testicular shrinkage, erectile dysfunction, and decreased libido. Additionally, about 40% of male users develop enlarged breast tissue due to steroids converting into estradiol.

Other side effects include a high prevalence of acne and increased risk of heart disease and stroke. While steroids can indeed enhance muscle mass and athletic performance, they come with a substantial set of health risks and side effects that must be carefully considered. The allure of rapid physical enhancement must be
weighed against the potential long-term consequences to health and well-being.

## Why do we get the munchies?

The munchies. It's that strong desire to eat everything in sight after you get stoned, even though you might have just had dinner. So why does this happen? And why does everything taste so good when you're high?
So first off, what is awesome is that scientists will actually get mice stoned to study them.
And recently there was research done where they got dozens of mice really high to try and figure out what caused the munchies
Turns out there's a set of neurons in your brain's hypothalamus that play a key role in controlling hunger, known as POMCs.
Researchers predicted that marijuana would decrease the activity in the POMCs because this is the area that makes you feel full. But they found the exact opposite. Getting high actually increase the activity in this part of the brain, but it's just releasing different chemicals.
So when you're not high, it's releasing chemicals that suppress your appetite, but when you get high, it's releasing chemicals that promote hunger. Thus, marijuana slips on the hunger switch in your brain.
One study found that marijuana decreased the gut hormone peptide Tyrosine tyrosine, which actually inhibits your food intake. But most importantly, pot increases the production of the hunger hormone known as ghrelin.
So the more ghrelin there is in your body, the

hungrier you are. But another reason you might want to chow down after you hit the bong is that. Food tastes and smells better when you're high.

No, seriously. In an experiment, researchers exposed mice to both banana and almond oil. So sober mice smelled the oil at first, but then stopped showing interest, a phenomenon known as olfactory habituation.

However, when mice were dosed THC, they kept sniffing and sniffing, showing an increased sense of smell. And marijuana also affects the glands located at the bottom of your mouth, which produce 70% of your saliva.

And they're called the submandibular glands. And so, when you are high, the THC actually binds to the glands, and the glands stop receiving messages from the parasympathetic nervous system, and therefore, you stop producing saliva.

And this is why you get pasties or cotton mouth or that famous dry mouth whenever you get stoned.

But don't expect all food to taste good. When we eat something delicious, it stimulates the release of dopamine, that feelgood chemical that's released and associated with the reward part of your brain.

And when you're high and eat something yummy, that amount of dopamine increases even further. However, it doesn't exactly enhance the taste of foods that you don't like, like bitter taste or something you find yucky.

Which is why, when you're high, you're probably going straight for the junk food or other things that
are already stimulating your dopamine reward center.

## The Science of Satiety: How Our Bodies Signal Fullness

Hunger is a compelling sensation, a primal call that demands attention. But equally intriguing is the process of feeling full, a complex interplay of physiological signals that tells us when to put down the fork. Understanding how our body knows when we're full involves a journey through the digestive system and into the intricate world of hormones and neural pathways.

As you indulge in a meal, the act of eating sets off the sensation of fullness. Food travels from your mouth down the esophagus to your stomach, gradually filling it. The stomach's muscular walls stretch to accommodate the incoming food, much like a balloon inflating. This stretching is detected by nerves entwined around the stomach, which then communicate with the brain via the vagus nerve, signaling that the stomach is filling up.

However, this physical expansion is just one piece of the puzzle. The body also relies on chemical messengers or hormones, produced by endocrine cells throughout the digestive system. These hormones respond to specific nutrients present in your gut and bloodstream, increasing as digestion progresses. They travel to the hypothalamus in the brain, a key area controlling food intake.

Over 20 gastrointestinal hormones play a role in regulating appetite. One such hormone is cholecystokinin, produced in the upper small intestine in response to food. It not only reduces the rewarding sensation of eating but also slows down food movement from the stomach to the intestines, enhancing the feeling of fullness. This mechanism explains why eating slowly often leads to feeling fuller compared to rapid eating.

As nutrients and hormones circulate in the blood, they prompt the pancreas to release insulin. Insulin, in turn, stimulates fat cells to produce leptin, another crucial hormone. Leptin interacts with receptors in the hypothalamus, which houses two neuron sets: one that generates hunger and another that suppresses it. Leptin inhibits the hunger-inducing neurons and stimulates those that suppress hunger, signaling peak fullness.

This intricate communication network involving hormones, the vagus nerve, the brainstem, and the hypothalamus ensures that the brain receives accurate signals about the body's state of fullness. Research has shown that certain foods, like boiled potatoes, are more effective in sustaining satiety compared to others, like croissants. Generally, foods rich in protein, fiber, and water are more satisfying.

However, this state of fullness is temporary. After a few hours, the body restarts its internal dialogue. The empty stomach produces hormones like ghrelin, which reactivates the hunger neurons in the hypothalamus, and the cycle of hunger and fullness begins anew.

Feeling full is a sophisticated response orchestrated by our body's response to food intake, involving a delicate balance of physical expansion, hormonal signals, and neural communication. It's a testament to the body's remarkable ability to regulate its needs, ensuring we eat just enough to nourish ourselves.

## The Pancreas: Your Body's Multitasking Health Coach

Tucked beneath your ribs lies the pancreas, an organ that functions much like a personal health coach for your body. This unsung hero plays a crucial role in both digestion and blood sugar regulation, ensuring your body operates at its best.

The pancreas is strategically located behind the stomach, perfectly positioned to aid in the breakdown of food. It produces a special digestive tonic composed of water, sodium bicarbonate, and various digestive enzymes. Sodium bicarbonate neutralizes stomach acid, allowing these enzymes to effectively break down food. Lipase targets fats, protease breaks down proteins, and amylase divides carbohydrates into energy-rich sugars, which are then absorbed into the bloodstream to nourish the body.

Simultaneously, the pancreas performs the vital task of controlling blood sugar levels. It accomplishes this through the hormones insulin and glucagon, produced by specialized cells known as the islets of Langerhans. Maintaining balanced blood sugar levels is critical; too much or too little can have life-threatening consequences.

Post-meal, when blood sugar levels typically spike, the pancreas releases insulin. Insulin facilitates the movement of excess sugar into cells for immediate use or storage and signals the liver

to reduce sugar production. Conversely, when blood sugar levels dip, glucagon is released, prompting cells and the liver to release stored sugars back into the bloodstream. This delicate balance between insulin and glucagon is essential for maintaining stable blood sugar levels.

However, a compromised pancreas can disrupt this balance, leading to diabetes. In this condition, impaired insulin production causes blood sugar to accumulate, potentially leading to hardened blood vessels, heart attacks, kidney failure, and strokes. Simultaneously, cells are deprived of the sugar they need for energy, and elevated glucagon levels exacerbate the issue by increasing blood sugar further.

The pancreas, like any good coach, cannot work alone. It requires our active participation in maintaining our health through conscious lifestyle choices. By understanding and supporting the pancreas's functions, we can better manage our overall well-being, ensuring this vital organ can continue to perform its essential roles effectively.

## The Frontier of Bone Regeneration: Growing Bones Outside the Body

The prospect of growing human bones outside the body is transitioning from science fiction to reality. To grasp this groundbreaking advancement, we must first understand the natural process of bone growth within the body.

In a developing fetus, most bones begin as flexible cartilage. Bone-forming cells, known as osteoblasts, replace this cartilage with a spongy mineral lattice composed of calcium and phosphate. This lattice hardens as osteoblasts deposit more minerals, endowing bones with their characteristic strength. While the lattice itself is lifeless, living tissues, including blood vessels and nerves, integrate into it through specialized channels, reinforcing the skeleton that performs vital functions like organ protection, movement, and blood cell production.

However, the initial formation is not sufficient for functional strength. According to Wolff's Law, bones strengthen in response to the stresses placed upon them. This adaptive process requires a balance of materials, managed by osteoblasts and their counterparts, osteoclasts, which recycle bone material.

In space, the absence of gravitational strain leads to a dominance of osteoclast activity over osteoblasts, resulting in bone mass loss. This principle also guides the body's remarkable ability to repair broken bones, reconstructing them

almost seamlessly.

When natural repair is insufficient, such as in cases of cancer removal, traumatic injuries, or genetic defects, traditional solutions like metal implants or bone grafts from donors have limitations, including infection risks and functional constraints. The ideal solution is to grow a bone from the patient's own cells, tailored to the precise defect.

This innovative approach involves harvesting stem cells from the patient's fat tissue and using CT scans to model the missing bone segment. The model, created via 3D printing or using decellularized animal bones, serves as a scaffold for the patient's stem cells. In a bioreactor simulating bodily conditions, these stem cells differentiate into osteoblasts and other cells, colonizing and remodeling the mineral lattice into living tissue.

A crucial aspect of this process is mimicking the mechanical stresses bones experience in the body, adhering to Wolff's Law.

The bioreactor achieves this by circulating fluids around the developing bone, prompting osteoblasts to increase bone density.

Within three weeks, this lab-grown bone, now vibrant with living cells, is ready for implantation. While human applications are still in the experimental phase, successful implementations in animals herald a promising future for this technology.

The ability to grow bones outside the body represents a significant leap in regenerative medicine, offering hope for more effective, personalized treatments for a variety of bone-related conditions. This advancement not only showcases human ingenuity but also opens doors to new possibilities in medical science.

**The Itch Factor:**

Itching, a sensation familiar to all, often strikes at the most inconvenient moments. But beyond its annoyance, have you ever wondered about the science behind why we itch? On average, a person experiences numerous itches daily, triggered by various factors like allergies, skin dryness, or even certain diseases. Sometimes, itches arise seemingly out of nowhere, or just from the mere mention of itching.

Let's delve into one of the most common itch triggers: bug bites. When a mosquito bites, it injects an anticoagulant to prevent blood clotting. This substance, mildly allergenic to us, prompts the release of histamine, causing capillaries to swell and facilitating an increased blood flow to bolster the immune response. This swelling is akin to the reaction caused by pollen in your eyes. Histamine also activates the nerves responsible for itching, explaining why bug bites are so itchy.

The exact mechanism of the itchy sensation is not fully understood, and much of our knowledge comes from studying mice. In these studies, researchers found that itch signals in the skin are transmitted via a subset of nerves associated with pain. These nerves produce a molecule that sends a signal to the brain, creating the feeling of an itch. Scratching provides temporary relief by causing a mild pain signal that overrides the itch.

But why do we itch? The prevailing theory suggests that our skin has evolved to be highly sensitive to touch as a defense mechanism against external threats. This sensitivity prompts us to automatically scratch and dislodge potential dangers like stinging insects or poisonous plants. Interestingly, we don't feel itching in internal organs like our intestines, which are not exposed to these external threats.

However, anomalies in the itch pathways can lead to excessive itching, impacting health. For instance, delusory parasitosis is a psychological condition where individuals believe they are infested with parasites, causing relentless itching. Phantom itching in amputees, where itching is felt in a limb that no longer exists, is another example. This occurs due to severe nerve damage, confusing the body's normal nerve signaling.

To treat such conditions, innovative methods are being explored. For amputees, mirror therapy, where the patient scratches the remaining limb while looking at its reflection, can trick the brain into feeling that the non-existent itch has been relieved. Researchers are also investigating the genetic factors involved in itching and developing treatments to block the itch pathway.

In literature, Dante Alighieri even depicted a section of Hell where the damned are tormented by eternal itching, illustrating the age-old recognition of this vexing sensation. Understanding and managing itching is not just a matter of comfort but also a window into the complex interactions between our nervous system and external environment.

# How stress can make you sick.?

Stress is a feeling we all experience when we are challenged or overwhelmed. But more than just an emotion, is a physical response that travels throughout your entire body. In the short term it can be advantageous, but when activated to often or for too long, your primitive fight or flight stress response not only changes your brain but also damages many of the other organs and cells in your body. Your adrenal gland releases the stress hormones cortisol, epinephrine, also known as adrenaline, and norepinephrine. As these hormones travel through your bloodstream, they easily reach your blood vessels and heart. Adrenaline causes your heart to beat faster and raises your blood pressure over time, causing hypertension. Cortisol can also cause the endothelium or inner lining of blood vessels, to not function normally. Scientists now know that this is an early step in triggering the process of atherosclerosis or cholesterol plaque build up in your arteries. Together, these changes increase your chances of a heart attack or stroke. When your brain senses stress, it activates your autonomic nervous system. Through this network of nerve connections, your big brain communicates stress to your enteric, or intestinal nervous system. Besides causing butterflies in your stomach, this brain-gut connection can disturb the natural rhythmic contractions that move food through your gut, leading to irritable bowel syndrome, and can increase your gut sensitivity to acid, making you more likely to feel heartburn. Via the gut's nervous system, stress can also change the composition and function of your gut bacteria, which may affect your digestive and overall health. Speaking of digestion, does chronic stress affect your waistline? Well, yes. Cortisol can increase your appetite. It tells your body to replenish your energy stores with energy dense foods and carbs, causing you to crave comfort foods. High levels of cortisol can also cause you to put on those extra calories as visceral or deep belly fat. This type of fat doesn't just make it harder to button your pants. It is an organ that actively releases hormones and immune system chemicals called cytokines that can increase your risk of developing chronic diseases, such as heart disease and insulin resistance. Meanwhile, stress hormones affect immune cells in a variety of ways. Initially, they help prepare to fight invaders and heal after injury, but chronic stress can dampen function of some immune cells, make you more susceptible to infections, and slow the rate you heal. Want to live a long life? You may have to curb your chronic stress. That's because it has even been associated with shortened telomeres, the shoelace tip ends of chromosomes that measure a cell's age. Telomeres cap chromosomes to allow DNA to get copied every time a cell divides without damaging the cell's genetic code, and they shorten with each cell division. When telomeres become too short, a cell can no longer divide and it dies. As if all that weren´t enough, chronic stress has even more ways it can sabotage your health, including acne, hair loss, sex dysfunction, muscle tension fatigue, irritability.

Your life and mind are always going to have stress. But what matters to your brain and entire body is how respond to that stress.